DATE

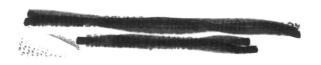

COMPACT *Research*

Hepatitis

Current Issues

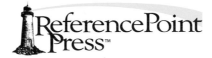

ReferencePoint Press™

San Diego, CA

Other books in the Compact Research series include:

Drugs
Alcohol
Antidepressants
Cocaine and Crack
Hallucinogens
Heroin
Inhalants
Marijuana
Methamphetamine
Nicotine and Tobacco
Performance-Enhancing Drugs

Current Issues
Abortion
Assisted Suicide
Biomedical Ethics
Cloning
The Death Penalty
Drug legalization
Energy Alternatives
Free Speech
Global Warming and Climate Change
Gun Control
Illegal Immigration
Islam
National Security
Nuclear Weapons and Security
Obesity
Stem Cells
Terrorist Attacks
U.S. Border Control
Video Games
World Energy Crisis

Diseases and Disorders
Anorexia
Meningitis
Phobias
STDs

Hepatitis

by Hal Marcovitz

Current Issues

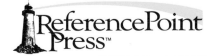

ReferencePoint
Press™

San Diego, CA

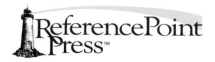

For more information, contact:
ReferencePoint Press, Inc.
PO Box 27779
San Diego, CA 92198
www.ReferencePointPress.com

LIBRARY OF CONGRESS CATALOGING-IN-PUBLICATION DATA

Marcovitz, Hal.
  Hepatitis / by Hal Marcovitz.
    p. cm. — (Compact research series)
  Includes bibliographical references and index.
  ISBN-13: 978-1-60152-039-5 (hardback)
  ISBN-10: 1-60152-039-5 (hardback)
  1. Hepatitis. I. Title.
  RC848.H42M37 2008
  616.3'623—dc22

                                               2007038874

Contents

Foreword

❝ Where is the knowledge we have lost in information? ❞

—"The Rock," T.S. Eliot.

As modern civilization continues to evolve, its ability to create, store, distribute, and access information expands exponentially. The explosion of information from all media continues to increase at a phenomenal rate. By 2020 some experts predict the worldwide information base will double every 73 days. While access to diverse sources of information and perspectives is paramount to any democratic society, information alone cannot help people gain knowledge and understanding. Information must be organized and presented clearly and succinctly in order to be understood. The challenge in the digital age becomes not the creation of information, but how best to sort, organize, enhance, and present information.

ReferencePoint Press developed the *Compact Research* series with this challenge of the information age in mind. More than any other subject area today, researching current issues can yield vast, diverse, and unqualified information that can be intimidating and overwhelming for even the most advanced and motivated researcher. The *Compact Research* series offers a compact, relevant, intelligent, and conveniently organized collection of information covering a variety of current topics ranging from illegal immigration and methamphetamine to diseases such as anorexia and meningitis.

The series focuses on three types of information: objective single-author narratives, opinion-based primary source quotations, and facts and statistics. The clearly written objective narratives provide context and reliable background information. Primary source quotes are carefully selected and cited, exposing the reader to differing points of view. And facts and statistics sections aid the reader in evaluating perspectives. Presenting these key types of information creates a richer, more balanced learning experience.

For better understanding and convenience, the series enhances information by organizing it into narrower topics and adding design features that make it easy for a reader to identify desired content. For example, in *Compact Research: Illegal Immigration*, a chapter covering the economic impact of illegal immigration has an objective narrative explaining the various ways the economy is impacted, a balanced section of numerous primary source quotes on the topic, followed by facts and full-color illustrations to encourage evaluation of contrasting perspectives.

The ancient Roman philosopher Lucius Annaeus Seneca wrote, "It is quality rather than quantity that matters." More than just a collection of content, the *Compact Research* series is simply committed to creating, finding, organizing, and presenting the most relevant and appropriate amount of information on a current topic in a user-friendly style that invites, intrigues, and fosters understanding.

Hepatitis at a Glance

Six Strains of the Disease

The six strains of the hepatitis virus are hepatitis A, B, C, D, E, and G. While hepatitis A, B, and C are most common in the United States, hepatitis is found on every habitable continent, infecting more than 500 million people.

Transmission

Hepatitis A is transmitted by oral contact with fecal matter. Hepatitis B and C are transmitted by contact with blood or other fluids of the body. Hepataitis D is spread by blood while hepatitis E is spread through contaminated water; both are rare in the United States. Hepatitis G, which only affects people already suffering from hepatitis A, B, and C, is transmitted by infected blood.

Main Symptoms

In all cases the virus attacks the liver. Symptoms of liver disease include jaundice—a yellowing of the skin and eyes—as well as fever, fatigue, stomachache, dark urine, light-colored stool, joint pain, nausea, loss of appetite, and vomiting.

Further Complications

Untreated, hepatitis can lead to cirrhosis, a scarring of the liver, as well as liver cancer. Each year some 6,500 Americans receive liver transplants; most are victims of hepatitis.

People Most at Risk

Most at risk for hepatitis A are toddlers who infect one another and the adults who change their diapers; for hepatitis B and C, intravenous drug users and gay men with multiple partners.

Epidemics

Poverty, war, and unsanitary conditions often cause epidemics. In the Darfur region of Sudan, a poor nation that has suffered through a bloody civil war, more than 1,700 new cases per month of hepatitis E were reported in 2004.

Controversies

Although nearly a third of America's 2 million prison inmates may be infected with hepatitis C, some corrections officials may be denying health care to many of them because of the high cost of treating hepatitis. Also, despite effective blood screening, the federal government does not permit gay men to donate blood out of fear they will spread hepatitis and other diseases. Gay men are among people most susceptible to contracting hepatitis B and C.

Vaccines

A vaccine for hepatitis B went into widespread use in 1986; all but 6 states mandate the immunization of young children. The hepatitis A vaccine has been available since 1995; it helped slash the infection rate by 82,000 cases a year.

Research Continues

While a search for the hepatitis C vaccine continues, scientists hope embryonic stem cells may be employed to grow new livers.

Overview

66 Hepatitis C mirrors America. It affects bus drivers, construction workers, even soccer moms. **99**

—Alan Brownstein, American Liver Foundation.

What Is Hepatitis?

Basically, hepatitis is an inflammation of the liver. The term stems from the Greek *hepar*, which means liver, and *itis*, which means inflammation. Inflammations of the liver can be caused by many common ailments, such as mumps and German measles, or by alcohol and drug abuse. However, a specific group of illnesses directly relate to the liver. Physicians identify them as hepatitis A, B, and C, the three most common forms. Other forms of the disease, which are identified as hepatitis D and E, are far less common in the United States but are still a concern to public health officials in America and elsewhere. Another form of the disease, known as hepatitis G, affects only patients who are already suffering from hepatitis A, B, or C.

The liver is one of the body's vital organs. Located on the right side of the body in the upper abdomen, the liver stores vitamins, sugars, and fats from food and uses them to manufacture chemicals such as proteins, which the body needs to function properly. The liver also manufactures bile, which assists in digestion. Finally, the liver breaks down and neutralizes substances that harm the body, such as alcohol. A person with a weak or damaged liver can experience jaundice, which is a yellowing of the skin and eyes, as well as fatigue, high fever, loss of appetite, vomiting, and muscle and joint aches. If left untreated, liver disease can lead to death.

Hepatitis A and the most common form of hepatitis B are treatable with drugs and in most cases will clear up within a few weeks or months. Hepatitis C is far more tenacious; drugs can control the symptoms, but the virus is likely to remain in the body for many years.

Acute or Chronic

Hepatitis can be acute or chronic. If the disease is contracted in its acute form, it will probably clear up after a short period of illness. In fact, many people will fight off the infection and never know they were ill. Hepatitis A is an acute form of the disease.

Chronic hepatitis may last a lifetime, although drugs can be effective in controlling the symptoms and may help prevent deterioration of the liver. Hepatitis B can be either acute or chronic, but most patients contract the disease in its acute form and are able to recover in a few weeks or months. Just 5 percent of hepatitis B patients develop the disease in its chronic form.

Between 20 and 50 percent of hepatitis C patients clear the virus from their bodies after a brief acute phase, but all other hepatitis C sufferers develop the illness in its chronic form. In fact, the disease lies dormant in the body for years or even decades before symptoms make themselves known. In the meantime, the disease damages the liver, and the damage is often irreversible. By the time the patients learn that they have contracted hepatitis C, they may be facing severe health issues. "Hepatitis C is an insidious disease," University of Texas Southwest Medical Center physician Willis C. Maddrey told *U.S. News & World Report*. "It creeps up on you."[1]

> " A person with a weak or damaged liver can experience jaundice, which is a yellowing of the skin and eyes, as well as fatigue, high fever, loss of appetite, vomiting, and muscle and joint aches. "

Victims of hepatitis range in age from very young children to older adults. Some well-known celebrities have contracted hepatitis, including actress Pamela Anderson, singers Naomi Judd and David Crosby, Congressman Joseph Moakley of Massachusetts, and Christopher Kennedy Lawford, the nephew of President John F. Kennedy. The death of baseball star Mickey Mantle was attributed to hepatitis C, which was aggravated by his long-time abuse of alcohol.

Unsanitary Conditions

Hepatitis is spread in many ways—through food, water, sexual contact, and sharing intravenous needles, among others—but in all cases a single cause is at the root: unsanitary conditions. In war-torn Iraq, the Baghdad neighborhood of Sadr City as well as the town of Mahmudiya reported hepatitis E outbreaks in 2004, caused by a breakdown of public sanitation. When sewage treatment facilities were damaged in the fighting, raw sewage pooled on the streets and was then tracked into homes. In Sadr City more than 150 cases of hepatitis E were reported, while in Mahmudiya more than 60 cases were reported. In the case of Pamela Anderson, the actress believes she contracted hepatitis C from her former husband, rock star Tommy Lee, after the couple received tattoos from the same needle.

> **Hepatitis is spread in many ways—through food, water, sexual contact, and sharing intravenous needles, among others— but in all cases a single cause is at the root: unsanitary conditions.**

Untreated sewage that is dumped in the ocean may carry hepatitis A; the virus can be picked up by shellfish, which if improperly cooked can pass the disease on to the people who eat them. Hepatitis A may also be spread by very young children: Fingers of infected children come into contact with the fecal matter in their diapers; then, they touch their playmates, who put their own hands in their mouths.

People who spend a lot of time around young children, such as day care workers, may also find themselves infected. Says physician James L. Achord, author of the book *Understanding Hepatitis*, "In one study of an epidemic, almost 15 percent of those sick with hepatitis were employees of or attended day care centers where the changing of diapers was a daily necessity. Children, not known for their inherent cleanliness, can easily pass the virus on to other children and to their parents, even when they themselves are not ill."[2]

How Prevalent Is Hepatitis?

The ancient Greek physician Hippocrates, who lived in the 5th century B.C., observed jaundice in his patients, suggesting that hepatitis has existed in the human population for at least 2,500 years. It was not until the 1940s, however, that medical researchers specifically identified the viruses hepatitis A and B. Hepatitis C was identified in 1988.

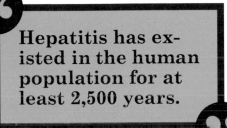

Hepatitis has existed in the human population for at least 2,500 years.

All forms of hepatitis are highly communicable, which means they spread easily. Hepatitis is found on every habitable continent on earth.

The U.S. Centers for Disease Control and Prevention (CDC) reports that as many as a third of all Americans have contracted hepatitis A in their lifetimes. In most cases they are able to recover without showing symptoms. Since they have thus experienced the disease, they are afterward immune.

As for hepatitis B, the CDC reports that about 60,000 new infections are reported each year. Most of those cases are in the acute form; however, about 1.25 million Americans suffer from chronic hepatitis B.

Hepatitis C is far more widespread. More than 4 million Americans have been infected. Hepatitis D and E are rare in America so the CDC does not compile statistics on sufferers.

Global Concerns

Efforts to stem the spread of hepatitis in the developing nations have been far less successful. In Africa, Asia, and South America, public sanitation is often neglected, vaccines are not readily available, and people receive little education about the disease and how it is spread. The World Health Organization (WHO), the public health arm of the United Nations, estimates that some 350 million people in the world suffer from the chronic form of hepatitis B, 170 million have been infected with hepatitis C, and 10 million suffer from hepatitis D.

In 2007 public health officials in Pakistan estimated that as many as 15 million of the country's 167 million citizens—nearly 10 percent of the population—had been infected with hepatitis B and C. The president of the Pakistan Society for the Study of Liver Diseases, S.M. Wasim Jafri, told the Lahore, Pakistan, *Daily Times*, "Our own research, along with those of other practitioners, shows that there is a large pool of 10 to 15 million hepatitis patients in Pakistan. These patients will infect others around them, initiating a vicious circle of disease of epidemical proportions."[3]

How Does Hepatitis Affect People?

Chronic hepatitis sufferers face long-term use of drugs to control their symptoms. Few hepatitis patients find the drug therapy a pleasant experience. The two main antiviral drugs for the treatment of hepatitis B and C, interferon and ribavirin, carry many side effects, including flu-like symptoms, weakness, and insomnia. (Sometimes the drugs are prescribed together, in a so-called drug cocktail.) One hepatitis C sufferer,

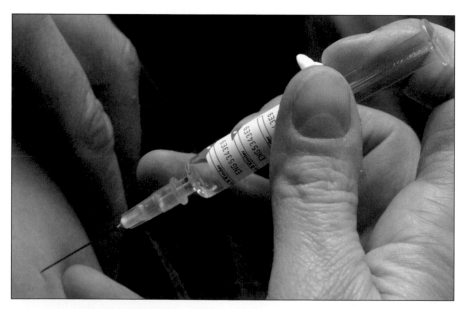

It is estimated that at least 1 million children have not received vaccines for many illnesses, including hepatitis B. Some health insurance plans have been dropping vaccinations as a covered expense, meaning people have to pay for the shots out of their own pockets—a sum that could total $400 or more per child.

Ohio fireman Ted Huffman, told *Newsweek* that interferon made him too weak to get out of bed, yet he often found himself incapable of sleeping. "I was a freakin' psychotic, suicidal mess,"[4] he told the magazine.

In many cases the drugs fail to achieve results. In 2005 the *Wall Street Journal* reported that just 50 percent of hepatitis C patients can expect the disease to go into remission after taking interferon and ribavirin for a year. What is more, in 2005, researchers at Queen Mary's School of Medicine and Dentistry in London, England, reported that some 80 percent of sufferers of hepatitis C are likely to develop the disease known as cirrhosis late in life. Cirrhosis is the accumulation of scar tissue in the liver, which prevents blood flow through the organ. When the liver becomes starved for blood, it is unable to properly carry out its functions. Cirrhosis sufferers face many health consequences, including liver failure and cancer.

> " Eighty percent of sufferers of hepatitis C are likely to develop the disease known as cirrhosis late in life. "

Each year about 6,500 people in America receive liver transplants, according to the American Liver Foundation. In addition, about 17,000 people are on the waiting list for a liver transplant. Most people who receive liver transplants are hepatitis patients.

Rising Death Rate

The death rate among hepatitis patients is expected to rise in the coming years, particularly for hepatitis C sufferers. That is because of the long-dormant aspect of the disease. Hepatitis C is spread when the blood of an infected person enters the body of a person who does not have the virus. For years the disease has been spread by intravenous drug needles, blood transfusions, and sexual activity, particularly among gay men with multiple partners. Since hepatitis C was not discovered until 1988, potentially tens of thousands of people who have contracted the disease do not know they have it, because the virus will lie dormant in their bodies for years or even decades.

In 2005 the CDC reported that the death rate in the United States for hepatitis C—at the time about 10,000 people a year—is likely to triple by 2015. One person who narrowly escaped death from the infection is Naomi Judd, who believes she contracted hepatitis C after being accidentally pricked by a used hypodermic needle while working as a nurse in the 1980s. When Judd was diagnosed with hepatitis C in 1990, doctors said she possibly had only three years to live due to liver damage. In Judd's case the drug therapy was successful, and she was able to resume her singing career. "Not only was my body poisoning me because of the hepatitis, but I was feeling like I had the flu from the interferon," she told the *Saturday Evening Post*. "It nearly pushed me over the edge. I was having trouble finishing my sentences, just disoriented."[5] As with Judd, many thousands of other people may be experiencing liver failure and not know it.

What Are the Social Impacts of Hepatitis?

In the United States and other industrialized nations, epidemics of disease are usually well contained. Gone are the days when an outbreak of a disease could kill thousands or even millions of people, which was the death toll of the flu pandemic that swept through the United States and Europe in 1918 and 1919. Quarantine signs routinely posted in the windows of scarlet fever patients or tuberculosis sufferers are also a thing of the past. Modern sanitation methods, drugs, and education have all served to contain widespread epidemics that formerly affected entire neighborhoods or communities.

> " The death rate among hepatitis patients is expected to rise in the coming years, particularly for hepatitis C sufferers. "

But in countries where little medical care exists, the impact of hepatitis can be devastating. Indeed, an outbreak of the disease can lead to an out-of-control epidemic and loss of life. In 2004 an epidemic of hepatitis E swept through the Darfur region of Sudan, which has suffered through a bloody civil war. The *Sudan Tribune* reported that during 2004 more than 1,700 new cases of hepatitis E had been reported per month in Darfur, dozens of which were lethal. Meanwhile, many people who escaped the civil war found shelter in the refugee camps of neighboring Chad. How-

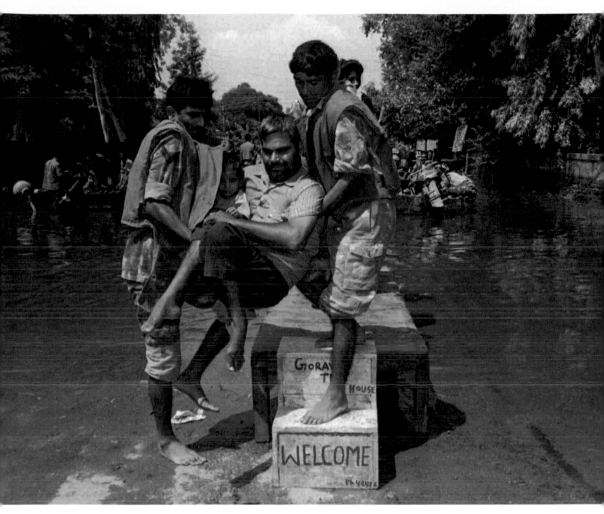

Flood victims are helped to safety by Indian soldiers. In 1955 the Yamuna River in India flooded, contaminating the drinking water of the city of New Delhi. The flood caused some 30,000 people to contract a form of hepatitis, later identified as hepatitis E.

ever, the squalid conditions in the camps led to an epidemic of hepatitis there as well.

Chad and Sudan have not been isolated cases. According to the WHO, hepatitis E outbreaks have occurred recently in more than 20 countries. And it does not take a war to spread the disease—sometimes a natural disaster can spread the virus. In 1955 the Yamuna River in India flooded, contaminating the drinking water of the city of New Delhi. The flood caused some 30,000 people to contract a form of hepatitis, later identified as hepatitis E.

Shame and Rejection

Diseases often place a social stigma on patients, and hepatitis sufferers are no exception. Chronic hepatitis sufferers face long-term and unpleasant drug therapies that have yet to show high rates of success. What is more, hepatitis patients may find little support among their friends, who may keep their distance out of fear for their own health. Clearly, the mental health of hepatitis patients will be tested during their therapies. Writing in the medical journal *Liver International*, physicians Edna Strauss and Maria Cristina Dias Teixeira report,

> Chronic liver diseases have a major impact on quality of life and can cause patients significant distress. . . . Chronic [hepatitis C]-related disease may cause a sense of stigmatization in the patient, leading to feelings of shame and rejection. It can also have a significant impact on social relations and self-esteem. The attention needed during clinical follow-up of patients and the use of antiviral medication in particular, create difficulties that can adversely affect both leisure and work activities even when patients are not receiving treatment. This overall picture reflects a disease that can compromise social relations and interfere with daily functions.[6]

> **Hepatitis patients may find little support among their friends, who may keep their distance out of fear for their own health.**

Hepatitis B carries an added risk for very young children. Pregnant women infected with hepatitis B may pass the virus on to their babies. Since pregnant women typically bleed during childbirth, it is possible that their babies may ingest a small amount of their mother's blood during delivery. Since babies cannot be vaccinated against hepatitis B while still in their mothers' wombs, the infants risk being born with the disease. If doctors are aware that the mother is infected with hepatitis B, her infant can be vaccinated within 12 hours of birth. That will enable the mother to breast-feed her baby, even if she does have the virus. If the baby's virus goes unchecked, it is likely he or she will become a hepatitis B carrier.

Controversies over Hepatitis

Professional tattoo artists have long been accused of spreading hepatitis by failing to sterilize their needles. Scientific studies that have examined the spread of hepatitis have largely exonerated the artists; indeed, medical researchers have not yet provided conclusive evidence suggesting that hepatitis can be linked to tattooing or body piercing.

> **An epidemic of hepatitis C has emerged in many American prisons.**

Still, medical professionals urge tattoo and body-piercing customers to use caution when they walk into a tattoo parlor and to seek assurances from the artist that he or she is using sterile equipment. Miriam Alter, the associate director for science at the CDC, told the *New York Times*, "Regardless of whether or not we can demonstrate that bacteria or viruses are spread in this manner, anything that pierces the skin and has blood on it can potentially spread an infection."[7]

Tattoos are very popular in American prisons, where amateur artists fashion needles out of Bic pens and make ink by grinding down the graphite in pencils. Hepatitis is also spread in prisons by inmates who engage in unprotected sex. As such, an epidemic of hepatitis C has emerged in many American prisons, meaning that county and state governments, which run most jailhouses, must shoulder the expense of treating inmates. A 2000 study by the U.S. Justice Department found that some 18,000 prison inmates have tested positive for hepatitis C.

Can Hepatitis Be Prevented?

The best way to make sure one never contracts hepatitis is to live in a clean environment, never have unprotected sex or abuse drugs, obtain the vaccinations that are available, and be wary of tattoo and body-piercing needles. But that does not mean a person can be totally protected from hepatitis or, in fact, from many other diseases. Accidental infections are always a danger. Natural disasters that can enhance the spread of the disease cannot be prevented. In the summer of 2005 Hurricane Katrina swept through Louisiana and Mississippi, displacing thousands of people from their homes and causing massive flooding on city streets. Sanitation systems were soon overtaxed. To escape from the danger, many people had to wade through flooded streets, where they risked contracting hepatitis as well as other ailments.

And yet, despite the danger, hepatitis was not regarded as a major health threat in the days following Hurricane Katrina. That is because the U.S. Health and Human Services Department rushed more than 50,000 doses of hepatitis A and B vaccines to the flooded areas within hours of the hurricane. There is no question that public health officials in America have responded well to the threat of hepatitis, which is why the rate of infections in the United States has declined in recent years. In 2007 the CDC reported that infections of hepatitis A had fallen 12 percent during the previous decade, which dropped the disease to its lowest rate in 40 years. Infection rates for hepatitis B and C also declined, the CDC said.

Eliminating Hepatitis

In America most states mandate the vaccination of children for hepatitis B. The CDC has also urged all states to mandate vaccinations for hepatitis A, but few states have adopted the agency's recommendations. According to the CDC, in addition to children, others who should be vaccinated for hepatitis A are people who travel to countries where infections are high, gay men with multiple partners, and drug abusers. Although research continues, at the present time there are no vaccinations available for hepatitis C, D, or E.

As such, it is not likely that hepatitis will soon be eliminated as a health risk in the United States or elsewhere in the world. Wherever poverty exists, conditions are usually ripe for the spread of hepatitis. In places where warfare rages, basic human services—including public sanitation—often break down, which can help spur an epidemic of the virus. In the years ahead physicians, political leaders, educators, and others will find themselves facing many challenges as they work toward controlling the spread of hepatitis.

How Does Hepatitis Affect People?

"My doctors tell me I won't die of liver problems. I'm one of the lucky ones."

—Roger Dillan, hepatitis C patient.

In the 1970s guitarist David Marks performed with such rock stars as the Beach Boys and Warren Zevon. He also partied hard, drinking heavily and using drugs. Two decades later, while still maintaining a busy schedule as a musician, he started feeling ill and was bothered by a pain in his side. "I had a hard time traveling," he told the *Times* of London. "I got tired easily. I was getting infections, I had more coughs and colds, and I got ill more than usual when I drank—my liver wasn't processing alcohol as well as it normally did."[8]

After seeing a doctor, Marks discovered that his ailments, including the pain he felt in his side, were due to an inflammation of his liver. Evidently, he had used a needle tainted with the hepatitis virus while abusing drugs. Marks eventually recovered from his bout with hepatitis, but it took several years before he could resume his music career. He was forced to take antiviral drugs that sapped his strength. "Yesterday, I slept for 14 hours," Marks told *Newsweek* in 2002. "My energy level is way low and there's a certain amount of depression. I find myself gazing into space."[9]

Common Strains

Marks was diagnosed with hepatitis C, one of six communicable forms of the disease. Each form of hepatitis is caused by a separate virus. The viruses may affect people differently, causing different symptoms. In fact, some people may be able to shake off the hepatitis virus without even knowing they have it; others, who contract the chronic form of the disease, may face long years of pain and suffering.

Hepatitis A is spread through contact with contaminated feces. The disease is often spread in places where dirty diapers are common, such as day care centers. Hepatitis A is contracted mostly by young children, who develop the acute form of the disease and therefore recover quickly with no long-lasting effects. However, the disease is also spread through fecal contamination of food, which can occur in restaurants where sanitation standards are low. Cooks whose hands are contaminated with fecal residue can spread the virus by handling food. That is why restaurants frequently post signs in their restrooms ordering employees to wash their hands before they return to work. Still, even in adults, hepatitis A usually clears up after a few weeks or months.

> " Some people may be able to shake off the hepatitis virus without even knowing they have it; others, who contract the chronic form of the disease, may face long years of pain and suffering. "

Hepatitis B is spread when blood, saliva, semen, or other bodily fluids from an infected person enter the body of a person who is not infected. That can occur through illicit drug use because drug abusers frequently share needles. Tattoo needles that are not sterilized between uses can also spread hepatitis B. People who share other personal items, such as razor blades or toothbrushes, can spread hepatitis B. Indeed, a razor blade that nicks the face or leg during a close shave or a toothbrush used against a bleeding gum could contain small traces of blood. The disease is also spread through sexual contact, particularly among gay men with multiple partners.

Hepatitis C is spread through contact with the blood of an infected person. As with hepatitis B, transmission can occur by sharing needles, razors, or other personal items that may contain the blood of an infected person. Hepatitis C can also be spread through sexual contact when bleeding occurs, most frequently among gay men who have multiple partners. Many people who received blood transfusions prior to 1990 contracted the disease because

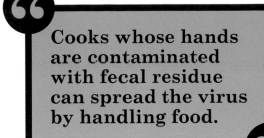

Cooks whose hands are contaminated with fecal residue can spread the virus by handling food.

until then a test that could detect hepatitis C in the blood of donors did not exist. Therefore, many people infected with hepatitis C may have donated blood. Since hepatitis C often lies dormant in the body for years or even decades, it is possible that many people who were infected with hepatitis C prior to 1990 are still not showing symptoms and are, therefore, not aware they are carrying the disease. Today, hepatitis C tests are administered to all donated blood.

Danger to Travelers

Hepatitis D and E are rare in America; nevertheless, Americans who travel in places where the diseases are common should be aware of the dangers. Hepatitis D is spread by blood and only affects people who are already infected with hepatitis B. Together, the two diseases are likely to lead to cirrhosis as well as other ills such as fluid in the abdomen and bleeding in the esophagus. Hepatitis E is spread through contaminated water and is most common in developing countries where people obtain their water from unsanitary supplies such as public wells or rivers. Like other forms of hepatitis, hepatitis E can lead to severe liver disease.

Hepatitis G affects only patients who are already suffering from hepatitis A, B, or C. The disease is transmitted by infected blood. It does not appear that the virus makes existing symptoms worse or causes new symptoms to occur in hepatitis patients. Hepatitis G is treated with the same drugs administered to patients who suffer from either hepatitis B or C.

During the 1990s a team of researchers thought they had discovered a new strain of the disease and labeled it hepatitis F. Subsequent tests revealed that the strain was no different from existing forms of the disease, thus, the designation "hepatitis F" was dropped.

Hepatitis A, B, C, D, E, and G are forms of viral hepatitis, spread by viruses that live in fecal matter, water, blood, or other bodily fluids. Another form of the disease, known as autoimmune hepatitis, is non-viral. It is extremely rare and is not spread from person to person. Auto-immune hepatitis occurs when the body's immune system attacks the liver. Doctors are not sure what causes autoimmune hepatitis; however, the symptoms and dangers of the disease are similar to viral hepatitis.

How the Virus Works

Doctors and scientists have been fighting viruses for hundreds of years. Among the most deadly viruses that have afflicted people are the small-pox, polio, rabies, and yellow fever viruses, as well as human immunode-ficiency virus, or HIV, which is the virus that leads to the disease known as acquired immune deficiency syndrome, or AIDS. Colds and the flu are also spread through viral infections. Most viruses, including the hepa-titis viruses, work in similar ways.

A virus is a microscopic parasite composed of organic chemicals and genetic material, which are the same materials that form the cells in animals and plants. However, viruses are not truly living organisms because they cannot survive on their own. They must attach themselves to living cells.

A hepatitis virus that enters the blood of an unaffected person will attach itself to a healthy cell and inject its genetic material into the cell. The cell, which naturally reproduces itself, will do so, only now it will produce cells infected with the hepatitis virus. Soon, the virus will take over the healthy cells and kill them, then move on to other healthy cells where the process will be repeated.

> "Many people who received blood transfusions prior to 1990 contracted the disease, because until then a test that could detect hepati-tis C in the blood of donors did not exist."

Most viruses attack parts of the body and produce symp-toms. A cold virus, for example, may leave the patient with a scratchy throat and runny nose for a few days. Before it was virtually wiped out through an effective vaccine, the polio virus attacked human nerves and muscles, often leaving its victims crippled.

The hepatitis virus attacks the liver, causing the organ to become inflamed and making it difficult for the liver to carry out its functions. Once a patient is afflicted with a failing liver, he or she may become jaundiced—a yellowing of the eyes and skin caused by the liver's failure to break down the bile that it manufactures. Other symptoms of hepatitis include fever, fatigue, stomachache, dark urine, light-colored stool, joint pain, nausea, loss of appetite, and vomiting.

Cirrhosis and Liver Cancer

When the liver is inflamed it often becomes scarred. Extensive scarring of the liver is known as cirrhosis, which can be a serious ailment in many hepatitis patients. When the liver becomes filled with scar tissue, blood flow to the liver is reduced. This condition makes it difficult for the liver to carry out its functions. For example, when blood is cut off from the liver, the remaining healthy blood vessels in the liver expand under pressure. This condition forces bile and other fluids out of the liver into adjacent places, such as the stomach. That is why hepatitis patients often suffer from fluid buildup in their stomachs.

> In the United States liver cancer is the fifth leading cause of cancer deaths, accounting for more than 400,000 victims a year.

Also, the blood must find another place to go. "When blood that normally goes through the liver and into the heart meets resistance, it will find an easier path," says physician James L. Achord. "One such path is through the small veins in the esophagus."[10] The esophagus is a tube that carries food from the mouth to the stomach. When the pressure in the veins that line the esophagus build up, they may rupture and start to bleed. That is why hepatitis patients may find themselves coughing up blood. If doctors cannot stop the bleeding, the condition may become life threatening.

Cirrhosis has also been found to be a precancerous condition, meaning that if the disease's progress is not arrested, cancer of the liver could result. In the United States liver cancer is the fifth leading cause of cancer

deaths, accounting for more than 400,000 victims a year. Most liver cancer is preceded by cirrhosis.

Can Hepatitis Be Fatal?

Certainly, hepatitis patients who develop cancer face the likelihood that
their diseases could become fatal. But most forms of hepatitis can also be
fatal long before they reach the cancerous stage.

Hepatitis A exists only in the acute phase, so the disease usually does
not progress to a fatal stage. Hepatitis B and C can be fatal, though.
According to the U.S. Centers for Disease Control and Prevention, as
many as 25 percent of chronic hepatitis B sufferers will succumb to the
disease, while hepatitis C will cause death in as many as 5 percent of
chronic sufferers.

The death of Peter Nowak provides a typical example. A victim of
a car accident in 1979, the advertising executive from Great Britain
received blood transfusions during an operation to save his badly injured
legs. Evidently, some of the blood provided to Nowak was tainted with
hepatitis C.

In 2001 he started feeling fatigued while also suffering from persis-
tent flulike symptoms. Then, his stomach swelled to the size of a football.
In 2005 he was diagnosed with hepatitis C. By that time his liver was so
damaged that it could not filter out the body's waste products. Every few
weeks doctors had to insert a tube known as a catheter to drain Nowak's
stomach. "He was going downhill in front of our eyes," Nowak's daughter, Kiri, told the *London Daily Mail*. "He started to look real pale and
skinny—almost not like Dad anymore."[11]

Just before Christmas in 2005, Nowak woke up with agonizing pains
in his stomach. His family decided to drive him to the hospital, but on
the way he lost consciousness. He died on December 29.

Liver Transplants

When Nowak died he was on a waiting list for a new liver. In America
some 17,000 people are waiting for liver transplants, and most of them
are hepatitis victims. According to the American Liver Foundation, about
6,500 liver transplants are performed each year.

Since everyone is born with a single liver, the only source of whole livers
for transplants is from deceased people. Typically, livers of people who die in

accidents or from head injuries are donated by family members. Sometimes, people do arrange in advance to be organ donors. Many states ask that applicants for driver's licenses state whether they wish to be organ donors; if they do, the words "organ donor" are printed on their licenses so that doctors know to harvest their organs soon after they are declared dead.

Because the number of people in need of new livers is far greater than the livers available from deceased donors, doctors have found that in some cases they can transplant a portion of a living person's liver into the body of a recipient. This procedure, known as a "living-related transplant," is usually limited to immediate family members because in such cases it is unlikely that the recipient's body will reject the donated portion. The portion that is donated then grows into a new liver; likewise, the portion that remains in the donor's body also grows back into a full liver.

> "Interferon, which must be injected, causes flu-like symptoms, headaches, fever, fatigue, loss of appetite, nausea, vomiting, depression, and hair loss."

How Is Hepatitis Treated?

Hepatitis A is not treated with drugs that specifically target the virus, although physicians may prescribe medications to ease the symptoms. The more serious forms of the disease, hepatitis B and C, are treated with antiviral drugs known to have limited success. Antiviral drugs are a relatively recent advancement; developed in the 1980s, they employ chemicals that block the protein molecules in the viruses that enable the diseased cells to reproduce themselves.

Typically, patients receive the drugs interferon and ribavirin for as long as a year. Some patients take one of the drugs; others are prescribed both drugs. Studies show that the drugs have a success rate of about 50 percent.

What is more, each drug has unpleasant side effects. Interferon, which must be injected, causes flulike symptoms, headaches, fever, fatigue, loss of appetite, nausea, vomiting, depression, and hair loss. Ribavirin can be taken in pill form. It causes severe anemia, which is oxygen-poor blood. People who suffer from anemia are often weak, fatigued, and unable to concentrate. Severe anemia can lead to heart failure. Ribavirin can also cause birth defects, which means it should not be taken by pregnant women. "The treatment is not fun," Eugene Schiff, liver specialist at the University of Miami School of Medicine, told *U.S. News & World Report*. "But we can cure the disease in about half the people. And I mean cure it."[12]

There is no question that hepatitis, in most of its forms, is an unpleasant disease that takes a mental and physical toll on its victims. In its chronic form, hepatitis causes pain, illness, and in many cases, death. Indeed, people who survive hepatitis regard themselves as incredibly lucky. Kenneth DeLisle, a minister from Winnipeg, Canada, endured the drug therapy and recovered from the disease. "Hepatitis is still a stress factor in my life," he told *Maclean's* magazine, "but it is just something I live with as opposed to something I worry about."[13]

How Does Hepatitis Affect People?

66 The liver has been variously described as the seat of the soul, the source of emotions, and a predictor of the future. It is the body's largest single organ and is necessary for life. 99

—James L. Achord, *Understanding Hepatitis.* Jackson: University Press of Mississippi, 2002.

Achord is professor emeritus at the University of Mississippi Medical Center and has written extensively on liver disease.

66 It makes me so angry to think of all those years Dad was walking around with this deadly virus, but was oblivious. 99

—Kiri Nowak, quoted in Olivia Holcombe, "The Secret Assassin," *Daily Mail* (London), February 20, 2007.

Nowak is the daughter of well-known advertising executive Peter Nowak, who died from a hepatitis C infection.

Primary Source Quotes

* Editor's Note: While the definition of a primary source can be narrowly or broadly defined, for the purposes of Compact Research, a primary source consists of: 1) results of original research presented by an organization or researcher; 2) eyewitness accounts of events, personal experience, or work experience; 3) first-person editorials offering pundits' opinions; 4) government officials presenting political plans and/or policies; 5) representatives of organizations presenting testimony or policy.

"Consider the risks if you are thinking about getting a tattoo or body piercing. You might get infected if the tools have someone else's blood on them or if the artist or piercer does not follow good health practices."

—U.S. Centers for Disease Control and Prevention, "Fact Sheet: Viral Hepatitis B." www.cdc.gov.

The U.S. Centers for Disease Control and Prevention is an agency of the federal government charged with monitoring public health risks.

"There are many more people who need a liver transplant than there are livers available for donation. . . . The waiting list is prioritized so the sickest people always go to the top of the list."

—American Liver Foundation, "Liver Transplant." www.liverfoundation.org.

The American Liver Foundation is a nonprofit organization that advocates for prevention of liver disease and helps raise money for scientific research.

"I was lucky I went into the hospital when I did because the virus was still in the early stages and I had minimal liver damage."

—David Marks, quoted in William Little, "The Day the Music Stopped," *Times* (London), March 16, 2005.

Former Beach Boys guitarist Marks most likely contracted hepatitis C by abusing drugs.

"When my liver could no longer function, the veins in my esophagus ruptured, causing me to vomit blood uncontrollably. . . . My crisis had moved me to the top of the donor list, and the next morning . . . I underwent my long-awaited transplant."

—Mitzi Miller, "A Lesson Before Dying," *Essence*, August 2007.

Miller, a victim of autoimmune hepatitis, received a liver transplant in 1998.

❝It's like having the world's worst case of the flu, the headache from hell, aching all over.❞

—Naomi Judd, quoted in Patricia Anstett, "Naomi Judd Offers Hope to Those with Disease," *Detroit Free Press*, June 19, 1998.

Judd, a country-and-western singer, was diagnosed with hepatitis C in 1990.

❝This study suggests that prolonged infection with hepatitis C leads to cirrhosis in the majority of those infected.❞

—Graham L. Foster, quoted in *Hepatitis Weekly*, September 19, 2005.

Foster, liver researcher at Queen Mary's School of Medicine and Dentistry in London, England, is the author of a study linking cirrhosis and hepatitis C.

❝The damage is so slow (in progression) that it takes years before you get sick enough to go to a doctor. So you are a carrier for a long time, unless you happen to have your blood tested.❞

—Dana Mortimer, quoted in Kristina Herrndobler, "Orange County Woman Shares Her Experiences with Hepatitis C," *Beaumont (TX) Enterprise*, December 26, 2006.

Mortimer is an Orange County, Texas, woman who contracted hepatitis C through a blood transfusion.

❝The development of symptoms [for hepatitis A] is directly related to the age of the person. The younger the person, the more likely the infection will be asymptomatic—without symptoms.❞

—Melissa Palmer, *Melissa Palmer's Guide to Hepatitis Liver Disease*. Garden City Park, NY: Avery, 2000.

Palmer is a liver specialist who practices in New York.

---

66 Always wash your hands with soap and water after using the bathroom, changing a diaper, and before preparing and eating food. 99

—U.S. Centers for Disease Control and Prevention, "Fact Sheet: Viral Hepatitis A." www.cdc.gov.

The U.S. Centers for Disease Control and Prevention is an agency of the federal government charged with monitoring public health risks.

---

66 Hepatitis C is a silent disease and can progress before you even know you have it. It is important to know the risk factors and avoid the disease. 99

—Susan Mayer, quoted in Michelle Mueller, "Hepatitis C: The Silent Epidemic," *Current Health* 2, January 2004.

Mayer is chief of pediatric gastroenterology at Yale University in New Haven, Connecticut.

How Does Hepatitis Affect People?

- According to the U.S. Centers for Disease Control and Prevention, **15 percent of hepatitis C cases** are transmitted through sexual contact, but only 3 percent are transmitted by monogamous partners.

- **Veterans of the Vietnam War** have a high risk for hepatitis C; many Vietnam veterans received battlefield blood transfusions before the virus had been discovered, and many also abused drugs during their tours of duty.

- By the 1960s the chance of contracting hepatitis C from a blood transfusion was **25 percent**; since the discovery of the virus and a method for testing it in blood, that chance has dropped to **0.001 percent**.

- Patients who suffer from autoimmune hepatitis often suffer from other autoimmune diseases, including **type 1 diabetes**, which attacks the pancreas; thyroiditis, an inflammation of the thyroid gland; colitis, an inflammation of the colon; vitiligo, a loss of skin color; and Sjögren's syndrome, which causes dry eyes and mouth.

- Hepatitis B or C patients who are **heavy consumers of alcohol** are more likely to be severely affected by the diseases, according to studies reviewed by the National Nurses Advisory Council for Liver Wellness and Viral Hepatitis.

The Liver and Its Functions

The liver, which is the largest organ in the body, has many functions. It produces bile, which aids in digestion. The liver stores vitamins, sugars, and fats the body draws from food and manufactures chemicals the body needs, such as proteins. The liver also helps remove impurities from the blood as it flows to the heart and returns clean blood to other organs in the body.

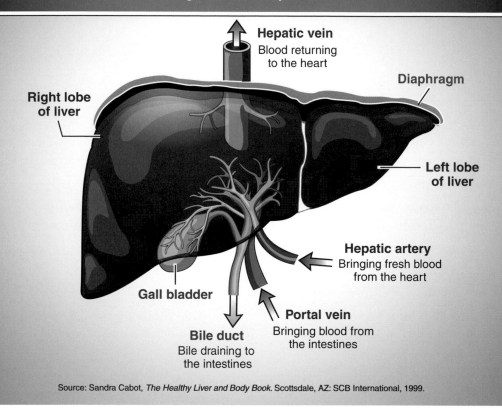

Hepatic vein
Blood returning to the heart

Diaphragm

Right lobe of liver

Left lobe of liver

Hepatic artery
Bringing fresh blood from the heart

Gall bladder

Portal vein
Bringing blood from the intestines

Bile duct
Bile draining to the intestines

Source: Sandra Cabot, *The Healthy Liver and Body Book*. Scottsdale, AZ: SCB International, 1999.

- **About 3 percent** of hepatitis B victims are unaffected by the symptoms but are unable to rid their bodies of the virus. They continue to be carriers and can infect others.

- About **75 percent of liver transplant patients** are still alive more than five years after their surgeries.

- Shellfish that live near places where sewage is dumped in the ocean can pick up and transmit hepatitis A. People who **eat raw shellfish**— including clams, oysters, and mussels—are at risk for contracting hepatitis A.

- Due to the spread of hepatitis C, demand for liver transplants in the United States is expected to **increase by 500 percent** between 2002 and 2008.

The Liver and Its Place in the Body

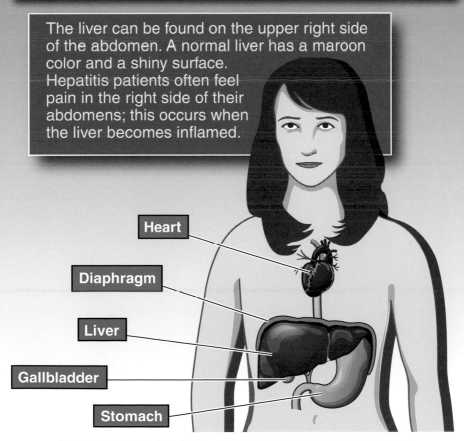

The liver can be found on the upper right side of the abdomen. A normal liver has a maroon color and a shiny surface. Hepatitis patients often feel pain in the right side of their abdomens; this occurs when the liver becomes inflamed.

Heart

Diaphragm

Liver

Gallbladder

Stomach

Source: Frank H. Netter, *Atlas of Human Anatomy,* 2nd ed., East Hanover, NJ: Novartis, 1997.

The Inflamed Liver

When a liver is afflicted with hepatitis it becomes inflamed, which means it becomes irritated and swells in size. This condition can cause significant pain to the patient. If the swelling is reduced within six months, the condition is regarded as acute, and the patient will not continue to suffer from symptoms. If the condition persists beyond six months, the patient has contracted a chronic form of hepatitis and is likely to face an extended period of unpleasant symptoms and complications that could include cirrhosis and liver cancer.

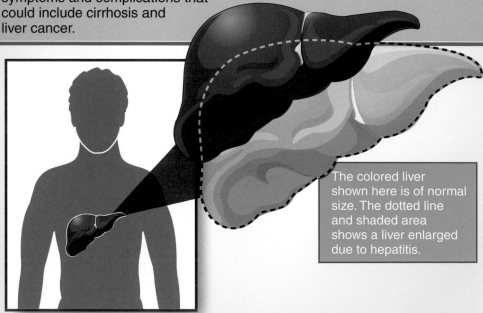

The colored liver shown here is of normal size. The dotted line and shaded area shows a liver enlarged due to hepatitis.

Source: *Encyclopedia of Health,* 3rd ed., Tarrytown, NY: Marshall Cavendish, 2003.

- The side effects of interferon and ribavirin, the medications used to treat hepatitis, are so severe that **20 percent of patients** chooses to give up the drugs rather than complete the therapy.

- Obesity can be a contributing factor in hepatitis cases; a 2008 Harvard Medical School study found that excess fat in the liver can make the symptoms of hepatitis more pronounced, leading to cirrhosis and cancer.

Cirrhosis and the Liver

Hepatitis can lead to cirrhosis, which is scarring of the liver. When the liver becomes full of scar tissue, it suffers from a lack of blood and cannot carry out its functions properly. A normal liver is shiny, but a scarred liver is marked with round lumps or knobs that can be as large as beans. When the liver starts failing, a patient may find bile forced into the stomach and blood forced into the esophagus. Cirrhosis is also regarded as a precancerous condition.

Normal Liver Anatomy Versus Stage Four Cirrhosis of the Liver

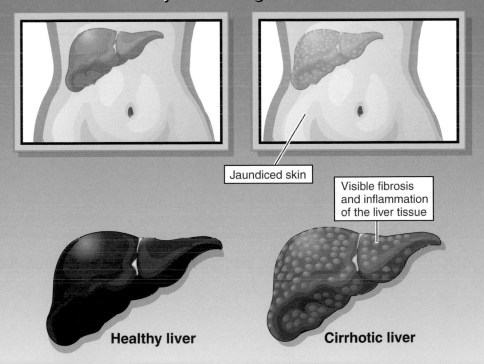

Jaundiced skin

Visible fibrosis and inflammation of the liver tissue

Healthy liver

Cirrhotic liver

Source: Edward Kiester Jr., editor, *The New Family Medical Guide.* Des Moines, IA: Better Homes and Gardens Books, 1982.

- Decades after the relationship between dirty needles and hepatitis was established, cases of hepatitis caused by unsanitary injections still surface; in 2002, a cancer clinic in Fremont, Nebraska, was closed by authorities after a nurse was found to be using old needles to administer injections. By the time the clinic was closed, 99 patients had been infected with hepatitis C.

How Prevalent Is Hepatitis?

> 66 If you used intravenous drugs even just a 'couple of times' decades ago, you may have acquired hepatitis C. Indeed, my patients are shocked to learn that something they experimented with in a most casual fashion twenty or twenty-five years ago could now be affecting their health. 99

—Sanjiv Chopra, Harvard Medical School.

Roots of the Disease

The ancient Greek physician Hippocrates wrote about a patient named Hermocrates, who came to him with high fever, inability to sleep, discolored urine, and jaundice—all symptoms of hepatitis. Hippocrates could do little for his patient but watch as the hepatitis racked the poor man's body. For nearly a month the Greek physician observed Hermocrates suffer. Finally, on the twenty-seventh day, the patient died.

Certainly, Hippocrates and the other early physicians who observed jaundice and the other symptoms in their patients did not know what caused them, nor did they associate the condition with liver disease. Slowly, though, medical science improved, and physicians and others started linking the symptoms together and formulating theories.

In the eighth century Pope Zacharias believed jaundice was infectious and suggested that people with the condition should be isolated from others. By the mid-1800s, physicians had chronicled several epidemics of jaundice, particularly in military camps—a highly logical conclusion, given the poor sanitation common in most army camps of the era as well as the abundance of bleeding wounds.

During World War II many Allied servicemen developed symptoms of hepatitis. Given the number of inoculations performed on soldiers as they headed overseas, military doctors concluded that they may have been infected while receiving vaccines for measles, yellow fever, and other diseases. A British doctor, F.O. MacCallum, first suggested that hepatitis is caused by a virus spread by human blood and that the servicemen who contracted the disease during the war received the virus when they were vaccinated with unclean needles that contained microscopic remnants of blood. In 1947 Mac Callum classified hepatitis into two types: hepatitis A, which he found was spread through food and water contaminated with fecal matter, and hepatitis B, which is spread through contact with contaminated blood and other fluids from the body.

> " A British doctor, F.O. MacCallum, first suggested that hepatitis is caused by a virus spread by human blood and that the servicemen who contracted the disease during the war received the virus when they were vaccinated with unclean needles that contained microscopic remnants of blood. "

Plague on Rural America

As bad as hepatitis has been in America, it could have been much worse. Starting in the early 1900s, American cities took steps to improve public sanitation and provide clean water to the public. City and state governments invested heavily in sanitary water systems as well as secure sewage disposal projects. The U.S. Pure Food and Drug Act of 1906 set very high standards for sanitation in the food-packing industries. Subsequent laws and infrastructure improvements have continued to ensure that food and water supplies in America are free of contamination.

Still, in the decades following those advancements many pockets of rural America lack adequate sanitation as well as access to health care and vaccines. Indeed, at one point during the 1990s, in some rural counties of Oklahoma, Arkansas, Missouri, South Dakota, Texas, New Mexico, Colorado, Arizona, Utah, Idaho, Nevada, California, Oregon, Washington, and Alaska, hepatitis A was very common. Those regions are home to large populations of American Indians and Native Alaskans, where remote reservations often lack adequate sanitary systems and the residents do not have easy access to vaccines or health care. A 2004 U.S. Centers for Disease Control and Prevention study found that during the 1990s, hepatitis A rates among some communities of American Indians and Native Alaskans were as high as 104 cases per 100,000 people—more than 50 times the national average. Public health officials reacted to the crisis and instituted a widespread hepatitis A vaccination program. In recent years infections in rural regions of America have declined dramatically, and now the infection rate among Native Alaskans and American Indians is believed to be below 2 cases per 100,000 people.

> **The spiraling cost of health care in America has also had a hand in helping to spread hepatitis as well as other infectious diseases.**

Common in Cities

People who live in inner cities often face similar public health dangers—mostly because of the rampant problem of drug abuse. Hepatitis B and C can both be spread through contact with unclean intravenous needles, a common occurrence among drug abusers, who frequently share their needles. Also, many cities are home to large populations of gay men who risk contracting hepatitis A, B, and C because of the nature of gay intercourse—anal sex without a condom may result in contact with blood and fecal matter. A 2006 study by the Chelsea and Westminster Foundation of London, England, found that a third of all gay men in London can be expected to contract hepatitis B by the time they reach 35. Tony Rodriguez, a gay physician from Philadelphia, told the *Advocate*, a magazine that reports on the gay community, "Gay men are especially at risk for hepatitis A and B because of their sexual practices. We need to get the word out."[14]

Even in middle-class or affluent communities, hepatitis can be a problem. Most states require children to be immunized for a variety of diseases, including hepatitis B, before they enter public schools. However, all but two states—West Virginia and Mississippi—allow parents to have immunizations withheld from their children on religious grounds. In addition, many states permit parents to have immunizations withheld from their children on philosophical grounds, meaning that parents may simply not agree with the government telling them how to live their lives. (That is not an unusual occurrence in society: In 2007 many parents balked when Texas mandated that all teenage girls receive vaccinations for human papillomavirus, a sexually transmitted disease that can lead to cervical cancer. Many parents objected out of fear that the vaccination could prompt their daughters to become sexually active.)

The spiraling cost of health care in America has also had a hand in helping to spread hepatitis as well as other infectious diseases. It is estimated that nearly 50 million Americans do not have health insurance. Mostly, these are unemployed people or working people whose employers do not provide health insurance as an employment benefit. Usually, state governments will step in and provide free vaccines to children, but in recent years states are finding they do not have the money to provide vaccines. It is estimated that at least 1 million children have not received vaccines for many illnesses, including hepatitis B. What is more, some health insurance plans have been dropping vaccinations as a covered expense, meaning people have to pay for the shots out of their own pockets—a sum that could total $400 or more per child. Pediatrician Grace Lee of Harvard Medical School told the Associated Press, "Health insurance plans are not necessarily keeping up with the new vaccines."[15]

> " According to the World Health Organization . . . , when compared with the rest of the world the infection rate for hepatitis in the United States is relatively low. "

Epidemics in Developing Nations

Hepatitis A, B, and C are not only common in the United States, they can be found elsewhere in the world as well. In fact, according to the World Health Organization (WHO), when compared with the rest of the world, the infection rate for hepatitis in the United States is relatively low. For example, according to the WHO, in Central America, South America, Africa, many countries of Europe and the Middle East, and large portions of Asia, "nearly all children are infected with hepatitis A before the age of 9."[16] Those same regions are also prone to high levels of hepatitis B and C. "In these areas, about 70 to 90 percent of the population becomes hepatitis B–infected before the age of 40,"[17] states a WHO report.

Typically, these countries in the developing world lack adequate public sanitation as well as access to vaccines, health care, and condoms. What is more, hepatitis D and E—virtually unknown in the United States—are common in many other countries. "Epidemics of hepatitis E have been found in much of Central and Southeast Asia, North and West Africa and Mexico, confined to geographic areas where fecal contamination of drinking water is common,"[18] states another WHO report.

> " Many victims of hepatitis C are paying now for the freewheeling lifestyles they led in the 1960s and 1970s—an era in which drug abuse and sexual freedom first found a wide and receptive audience among young people in America. "

Who Is Most at Risk?

Clearly, just about anyone can contract hepatitis if they are not careful. Travelers to countries where hepatitis D and E are common must be careful to observe a high level of personal hygiene and only eat foods and drink liquids they are sure are free of contamination.

In America, among the people most likely to contract forms of the disease are family members of infected people. Just living in the same house as an infected person can place somebody at risk. Therefore, brothers and sisters or sons and daughters of hepatitis victims must be careful not to mistakenly pick up the wrong toothbrush or shave with the same razor used by the hepatitis sufferer. An innocent game of roughhousing in the backyard is out of the question—any injury that results in a cut can produce blood, which is a transmitter of hepatitis B and C.

Hepatitis A can be contracted just about anywhere in the United States. Children are most susceptible, but adults can get it, too—particularly gay men with multiple partners who do not use condoms, and people who travel to other countries where hepatitis A is common. Usually, the symptoms will start showing up within two to six weeks of contracting the disease.

Likewise, hepatitis B can also be sexually transmitted, particularly among gay men with multiple partners. Hepatitis B is also common among intravenous drug abusers. Hepatitis B patients are likely to start feeling ill between five weeks and six months after contracting the disease.

> " Public health officials fear that young people are ignoring warnings about abusing intravenous drugs, the result of which could be contracting hepatitis C. "

As with hepatitis B, hepatitis C is also transmitted through sexual contact as well as intravenous drug abuse. Unlike hepatitis B, though, it could take years or even decades before hepatitis C victims start showing symptoms. That is why many victims of hepatitis C are paying now for the freewheeling lifestyles they led in the 1960s and 1970s—an era in which drug abuse and sexual freedom first found a wide and receptive audience among young people in America.

Hepatitis C's Victims

Unlike hepatitis A and B, which were identified in 1947, it was not until 1988 that researchers identified the virus that causes hepatitis C. Until then, doctors were stumped by the ailment—their patients were showing all the symptoms of liver disease, but their bodies lacked the hepatitis A or B viruses. In fact, before the hepatitis C virus was finally identified, doctors called the disease "non-A, non-B hepatitis."

The virus was identified by scientists at Chiron Corporation, a biotechnology company that specializes in blood screening tests. Biochemists Michael Houghton, Qui-Lim Choo, and George Kuo identified the virus by studying its genetic makeup.

Before the breakthrough, though, the virus was unknown, so hospitals and other organizations that accept blood donations could not test for the virus in donated supplies. That is why many victims of accidents, criminal acts, battlefield wounds, and other incidents were infected with hepatitis C when they received blood transfusions during their treatments. Among the most unfortunate victims of hepatitis C were hemophiliacs, who may receive many transfusions because their blood's lack of a natural clotting factor often results in uncontrollable bleeding. According to the CDC, before a blood test was developed for hepatitis C, virtually the entire population of hemophiliacs in America and other countries was infected with the disease.

Among the other victims of hepatitis C are those former flower children from the 1960s or disco denizens from the 1970s who shared needles and are finding out now that they contracted hepatitis C in those carefree days. Indeed, even the 1970s partyers who eschewed injected drugs for cocaine, which they thought would be a safer alternative, have found that that is not necessarily the case. Cocaine is sniffed through a straw or tube—often a rolled-up dollar bill. The drug irritates the inside of the nose, often causing slight bleeding. Tiny droplets of blood may be left as residue on the dollar bill as it is passed around the table, then ingested by the next cocaine sniffer.

One of the most famous drug abusers of the 1960s and 1970s is David Crosby, a founder of the rock group Crosby, Stills & Nash, which performed at the Woodstock rock festival in 1969. In the early 1990s Crosby was diagnosed with hepatitis C. In 1994 he received a transplanted liver. Emmet Keefe, a professor of medicine at Stanford University in California, told *U.S. News & World Report*, "These are [now] solid citizens who just played around in the late '60s and early '70s."[19]

New Epidemic Among Teens

But one does not have to be a child of the 1960s or 1970s to contract hepatitis C. Indeed, public health officials fear that young people are ignoring warnings about abusing intravenous drugs, the result of which could be contracting hepatitis C. The recent popularity of methamphetamine—which can be injected—is causing concern among health professionals. What is more, because of the popularity of piercings and tattoos, many teens risk contracting hepatitis C because they are not being careful about where they obtain their body art. And some young athletes looking for a shortcut in building up their bodies have taken anabolic steroids, which must be injected with intravenous needles. Sharing these needles can also spread hepatitis.

A study performed by the Massachusetts Department of Public Health found that between 2001 and 2005, the hepatitis C case rate tripled among young people between the ages of 15 and 25. (In 2001, 254 cases were reported; 4 years later, 784 cases were reported.) Maureen Jonas, a pediatric liver specialist at Children's Hospital in Boston, told the *Boston Globe*, "I am seeing, sadly, a fair number of 13-, 14-, 15-, 16-year-olds with intravenous drug use and hepatitis C. A lot of them—not all of them—knew that the person whose needle they shared had hepatitis of some sort. They just have a typical adolescent frame of mind that 'it's not going to happen to me.'"[20]

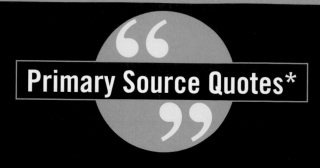

How Prevalent Is Hepatitis?

66 **Any type of needle that has been used by a person with hepatitis C can infect another person if it is used again without being sterilized properly.** 99

—Sanjiv Chopra, *Dr. Sanjiv Chopra's Liver Book*. New York: Pocket Books, 2001.

Chopra is a liver specialist and associate professor of medicine at Harvard Medical School in Massachusetts.

66 **Hepatitis B is one of the major diseases of mankind and is a serious global public health problem.** 99

—World Health Organization, "Fact Sheet on Hepatitis B." www.who.int.

The World Health Organization is the public health arm of the United Nations.

66 **Parents should be aware that withholding vaccinations leaves their child vulnerable to vaccine-preventable diseases in the event of an outbreak.** 99

—U.S. Centers for Disease Control and Prevention, *Immunization Laws*. www.hhs.gov.

The U.S. Centers for Disease Control and Prevention is an agency of the federal government charged with monitoring public health risks.

* Editor's Note: While the definition of a primary source can be narrowly or broadly defined, for the purposes of Compact Research, a primary source consists of: 1) results of original research presented by an organization or researcher; 2) eyewitness accounts of events, personal experience, or work experience; 3) first-person editorials offering pundits' opinions; 4) government officials presenting political plans and/or policies; 5) representatives of organizations presenting testimony or policy.

“Tommy [Lee] has the disease and never disclosed it to me during our marriage.”

—Pamela Anderson, quoted in *Toronto Star*, “Pamela Anderson Has Hepatitis C,” March 31, 2001.

Anderson, the former star of the TV series *Baywatch*, believes she contracted hepatitis C after receiving a tattoo from the same needle used to provide a tattoo for her former husband, rock drummer Tommy Lee.

“Because of its high fatality rate, AIDS is far more feared. However, worldwide, more people are made ill or die as a consequence of hepatitis B infection.”

—Baruch S. Blumberg, “Australia Antigen and the Biology of Hepatitis B,” *Science*, 1977, reprinted in Arien Mack, ed , *In Time of Plague: The History and Social Consequences of Lethal Epidemic Diseases*. New York: New York University Press, 1991.

Blumberg, a physician and biochemist, won the Nobel Prize in Physiology or Medicine for research that led to the discovery of a vaccine for hepatitis B.

“The actual number of infections (of hepatitis A) is difficult to estimate because the majority of people affected [do not show symptoms], do not become jaundiced, and therefore go undiagnosed. Such individuals serve as a reservoir of the virus and source of infection for others.”

—James L. Achord, *Understanding Hepatitis*. Jackson: University Press of Mississippi, 2002.

Achord is professor emeritus at the University of Mississippi Medical Center and has written extensively on liver disease.

“These viruses are shed in the feces of the infected person, and are then transmitted to another person via ingesting by mouth a small amount of infected stools. While such an occurrence may sound absurd, it is actually fairly common, especially in areas where poor sanitation is widespread.”

—Melissa Palmer, *Melissa Palmer's Guide to Hepatitis Liver Disease*. Garden City Park, NY: Avery, 2000.

Palmer is a liver specialist who practices in New York.

❝The majority of my patients experimented with drugs in the '60s and '70s and now work on Wall Street.❞

—Robert S. Brown, quoted in Paul Davies, "Long-Dormant Threat Surfaces: Deaths from Hepatitis C Are Expected to Jump," *Wall Street Journal*, March 31, 2005.

Brown is medical director of the Center for Liver Disease and Transplantation at New York Presbyterian Hospital.

❝I was always beat and scratched up and covered with somebody else's blood. The stuff showered off. I never thought it was a big deal. I thought I was tough.❞

—Ted Huffman, quoted in Geoffrey Cowley, Karen Springen, Anne Underwood, Nadine Joseph, Joan Raymond, and John Horn, "Hepatitis C: The Insidious Spread of a Killer Virus," *Newsweek*, April 22, 2002.

Huffman, a fireman from Euclid, Ohio, believes he contracted hepatitis C by coming into contact with victims of fires and accidents whom he carried to safety.

❝We tell people who have a partner with hepatitis C to use condoms.❞

—Ian Williams, quoted in Betsy Querna, "Emerging Epidemic," *U.S. News & World Report*, March 13, 2006.

Williams is chief of epidemiology for the CDC's Division of Viral Hepatitis.

❝I see a lot of successful people [with hepatitis] leading fulfilled lives: lawyers, business people, academics. The skid-row junkie is the kind of [typical hepatitis] sufferer in some cases but certainly isn't in many others.❞

—William Rosenberg, quoted in William Little, "The Day the Music Stopped," *Times* (London), March 16, 2005.

Rosenberg is professor of medicine at the University of Southampton in England and author of a study on the spread of hepatitis C in Great Britain.

Facts and Illustrations

How Prevalent Is Hepatitis?

- **Chimpanzees** can also contract the hepatitis C virus—mostly by bloodying one another in squabbles.

- Woodchucks can also contract the hepatitis B virus. The disease is responsible for causing **100 percent** of liver cancer cases in woodchucks; in humans, hepatitis B causes about **90 percent** of all liver cancer cases.

- More than **50 teenagers** in the Romanian village of Lungani were diagnosed with hepatitis A in 2007; health officials suspected lax personal hygiene was the cause.

- The *Journal of the American Medical Association* reported in 2007 that hepatitis B is a leading cause of illness and death in China; **nearly 10 percent of the country's population** of 1.3 billion people is infected with the chronic form of the disease.

- According to the U.S. Centers for Disease Control and Prevention, **66 percent** of hepatitis C sufferers in America are white and male, were born after 1945, and live above the poverty line.

Hepatitis Infections Worldwide

Hepatitis A and B are regarded as public health threats in the United States, but when compared with the rest of the world, the rate of infection in America is relatively low. According to statistics compiled by the World Health Organization, in parts of Africa, Asia, and South America, the rate of hepatitis B infection is greater than 8 percent of the populations. Meanwhile, the WHO

Hepatitis A Infections

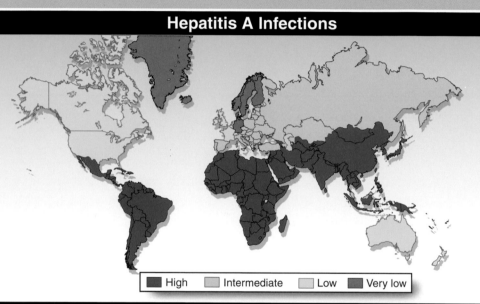

High   Intermediate   Low   Very low

Hepatitis B Infections

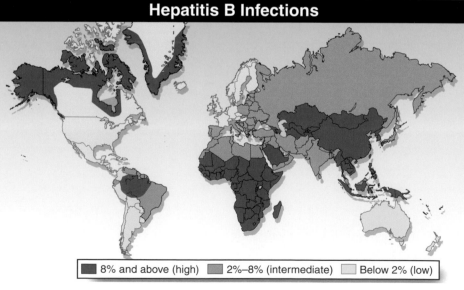

8% and above (high)   2%–8% (intermediate)   Below 2% (low)

also reports that the spread of hepatitis A is also low in the United States and other industrialized nations, while it is very high in South America, Africa, and Asia. As for hepatitis C, though, WHO statistics indicate the disease is more common in the United States than in some parts of Central and South America, Africa, and Asia.

Hepatitis C Infections

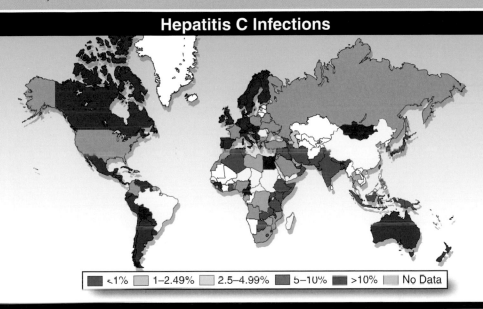

| ■ <1% | □ 1–2.49% | □ 2.5–4.99% | ■ 5–10% | ■ >10% | □ No Data |

Source: World Health Organization, Department of Communicable Disease Surveillance and Response. www.who.int.

- **Hepatitis E is spread through water infected with fecal matter**. Most outbreaks occur in developing countries where flooding is common following monsoon rains, which contaminate well water and strain the ability of sewage treatment plants to sanitize wastewater. Recent outbreaks have been reported in Algeria, Bangladesh, Borneo, China, Egypt, Ethiopia, Greece, India, Indonesia, Iran, Cote d'Ivoire, Jordan, Libya, Mexico, Myanmar, Nepal, Nigeria, Pakistan, Russia, Somalia, Sudan, and Gambia.

- Drug companies earn more than **$2.4 billion a year** manufacturing the vaccines for hepatitis A and B; in recent years the market has been growing at a rate of about 25 percent per year.

Hepatitis A and B on the Decline

Due to the availability of vaccines, the rates of infection for hepatitis A and B have fallen dramatically in recent years. In 2004, fewer than 6,300 cases of hepatitis B were reported, while hepatitis A cases numbered fewer than 5,700. Hepatitis B cases hit a peak in 1990, which was shortly after the vaccine for the disease became widely available. Hepatitis A cases also peaked in 1990 – years before a vaccine was developed. The statistics for hepatitis B are based on acute cases, only because the U.S. Centers for Disease Control and Prevention does not compile statistics on chronic hepatitis B cases; however, since all hepatitis cases begin as acute cases, the statistics provide a good indication of the decline of the disease.

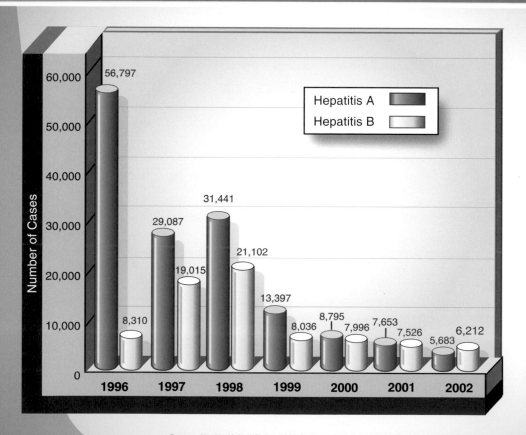

Source: *Health, United States 2006,* National Center for Health Statistics. www.cdc.gov.

A Sexually Transmitted Disease

Hepatitis is a sexually transmitted disease; statistics compiled by the U.S. Centers for Disease Control and Prevention in 2003 show that 15 percent of the patients who contract hepatitis C in the U.S. get the disease from their sex partners. In addition, statistics compiled between 1990 and 2000 by the CDC indicate that 10 percent of hepatitis A patients are gay men who have multiple partners, while another 14 percent of the patients contract the disease from their sex partners or others in their households.

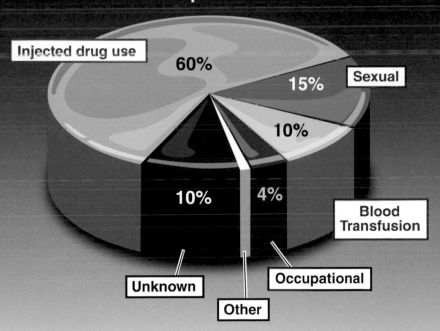

Sources of Hepatitis C Infections

Injected drug use — 60%
Sexual — 15%
10%
Blood Transfusion
10% — Unknown
4% — Other
Occupational

Source: U.S. Centers for Disease Control, *Hepatitis C and Viral Hepatitis, Historical Perspective*. www.cdc.gov.

- Hepatitis C is found in many people over the age of 60 in Italy and Japan. In one Italian village, World Health Organization researchers found an **infection rate of more than 33 percent**. The WHO concluded that from the 1950s to 1970s, doctors and dentists in Italy and Japan routinely reused intravenous needles, evidently without sterilizing them.

- The number of hepatitis C infections reached some **240,000 per year** during the 1980s. In 1990 a test was developed to screen donated blood for the hepatitis C virus. By 2004 the number of new infections for hepatitis C had dropped to about **26,000 per year**.

- In 1980, 10 teenagers in New Bern, North Carolina—among them the sons and daughters of some of the community's most affluent families—**died from hepatitis B infections**. A CDC investigation determined that the teenagers had been **abusing cocaine through intravenous injections** and were evidently sharing needles.

- Egypt is believed to have the **highest rate of hepatitis C** in the world. The WHO believes the high rate of hepatitis C in Egypt is due to the use of unclean needles for the injection of drugs used to treat diseases spread by parasitic flatworms.

What Are the Social Impacts of Hepatitis?

"What we need to do is turn hep C into just another disease—like heart disease, like diabetes, like cancer, so people don't have to deal with discrimination."

—Helen Tyrrell, chief executive of the Australian Hepatitis Council.

Suffering Alone

Despite its long history of afflicting people, hepatitis in all its forms remains a little-understood disease. For example, during the early 1980s when "non-A, non-B" hepatitis was first coming to the attention of physicians, many public health officials suggested that the disease was linked to the virus that causes AIDS. As such, they argued, the victims of "non-A, non-B" hepatitis were mostly gay men—an assumption that was eventually proven wrong.

Certainly, physicians have a better understanding now of hepatitis, but most everyone else harbors fears and misconceptions. "There is still so much misunderstanding about how it can be caught and how it affects people," Louise Chisholm, the head of a hepatitis C support group in Scotland, told the *Glasgow Herald*. "Hepatitis C can be very serious and may lead to liver failure, yet most people with it can still lead long and healthy lives."[21]

Even so, there is no question that hepatitis sufferers often find themselves facing the illness alone—a circumstance made even more painful because the disease can rob them of their energy, forcing them to stay at home for long periods. Their friends, fearing infection, no longer drop by to see them. Their family members may also keep their distance. Wrote physicians Edna Strauss and Maria Cristina Dias Teixeira in the medical journal *Liver International*, "People who live with the carrier suffer from fear of being infected with a potentially serious disease. In view of this, it is hardly surprising that patients infected with [the AIDS virus] or hepatitis C suffer more prejudice and feel more stigmatized than patients with other chronic diseases."[22]

Mental Anguish

When patients with potentially fatal diseases are isolated from others and forced to take drugs that make them feel ill, they often fall into the depths of severe depression. Depression is a mental illness characterized by feelings of sadness, hopelessness, and inadequacy. The illness often afflicts hepatitis patients. Naomi Judd told the *Detroit Free Press* that after her diagnosis, she suffered from depression. The mental anguish was so severe, Judd said, that she found herself unable to rise from bed in the morning. She said, "When you are told by medical authorities you have three years on this planet, that you're going to be taking a six-foot dirt nap, and that this is an absolutely incurable terminal illness, the sense of entrapment is so suffocating, so claustrophobic. It felt like there was no way out, like being buried alive."[23] Judd defied her doctors' predictions and recovered from hepatitis C; she also recovered from depression by taking antianxiety drugs.

Another hepatitis C sufferer, Lisa Waller of Sydney, Australia, told the *Australian* newspaper that her mental anguish went far beyond depression. Instead of hiding in her own world, unable to rise from bed or commu-

> **Hepatitis sufferers often find themselves facing the illness alone—a circumstance made even more painful because the disease can rob them of their energy, forcing them to stay at home for long periods.**

nicate with others, Waller found herself lashing out at friends and family members. Waller said the virus wore her down—she could not go for a walk without finding places to rest along the way. As for the drug therapy, Waller was forced to take weekly doses of interferon, which caused several side effects that also took a physical toll. "It was also the accumulated effect of all the minor things that can get you down," she told the *Australian*. "I had a

> When patients with potentially fatal diseases are isolated from others and forced to take drugs that make them feel ill, they often fall into the depths of severe depression.

lot of mouth ulcers. You lose your hair gradually, because it's a low dose (of interferon) over a long time, and you also don't feel particularly well. And I didn't get depression, but I did suffer from incredible rages."[24]

Effect on Women

Hepatitis can have a harsh impact on women, particularly if they are mothers or soon to be mothers. Infants born to mothers infected with hepatitis B and C are at risk for contracting the disease during childbirth. In their study, Strauss and Teixcira found that women who suffer from hepatitis C report higher degrees of mental anguish than do men, mostly because they fear infecting other family members. And since there is no vaccine for hepatitis C, infected mothers-to-be harbor a true fear of passing the disease on to their babies.

Women are also the primary victims of autoimmune hepatitis. Although the disease is rare—usually occurring in less than 200 cases per 1 million people—some 70 percent of all victims are women, particularly women between the ages of 15 and 40. Medical researchers do not know why women are afflicted with autoimmune hepatitis more so than men, although they suspect the malady is genetic—there is something about the chemical makeup of women's DNA that makes them more prone to be afflicted with autoimmune hepatitis.

The disease is not caused by a virus but by an attack on the liver waged by the body's immune system. The disease is treated not by interferon or ribavirin but by drugs that deaden the immune system, which slows the progression of the disease. Still, autoimmune hepatitis can be mistaken for viral hepatitis because the damage to the liver is similar. Stanley M. Finger, a chemistry professor at Johns Hopkins University in Baltimore, Maryland, told the magazine *Scientist* that his daughter's affliction with autoimmune hepatitis had a devastating effect on his family.

> "When she was 19, my oldest daughter was diagnosed with autoimmune hepatitis. As a family, we faced great stress and financial impacts. First, my wife quit work to care for our daughter until she was strong enough to return to college six months later. Moreover, insurance covered only part of my daughter's visits to specialists and the cost of [drugs]. We were fortunately able to absorb these financial impacts, but they can easily overwhelm a family."[25]

Financial Strain

The financial strain on victims of viral hepatitis is no less dramatic. Treatments of interferon and ribavirin can cost $20,000 or more a year. Americans with health insurance are fortunate because their plans may pick up some or all of the cost; Americans without health insurance will obviously find the cost staggering.

But the cost of living with hepatitis C does not end with the cost of the drug therapy. Hepatitis patients are often ill for months and unable to work; their families suffer because of loss of income. Students may miss months of school. The frequent trips to hospitals, physicians' offices, clinics, and other medical providers take enormous amounts of time; other family members may have to miss work to accompany the victims, who may be too weak or ill to transport themselves. In 2002 the White House Office of National Drug Control Policy estimated that it cost $312 million a year to treat hepatitis B and C patients in the United States. That number actually had dropped since 1992, when the agency estimated the cost at $462 million. With far fewer victims now of hepatitis C—due mostly to blood screening tests initiated in 1990—it should not come as a surprise that the annual cost of treating the disease has decreased. Nevertheless, hundreds of millions of dollars are still being spent each year by victims, their families, insurance companies, health care providers, and taxpayers, who must fund the treatments for hepatitis victims who live below the poverty line.

Tattoo Artists Defend Their Craft

Tattoo and body-piercing professionals have long shouldered accusations that they are responsible for spreading hepatitis B and C in the United States and elsewhere, since the needles they use in their craft often draw blood. Scientific studies have not provided conclusive evidence that the tattoo and body-piercing industry is responsible for spreading hepatitis infections. In 2005 the U.S. Centers for Disease Control and Prevention released a study assessing the spread of hepatitis C among nearly 8,000 college students in Texas who said they had received tattoos or piercings in parts of their bodies other than their earlobes. The study found that the rate of hepatitis C among those students was no higher than the rate found in the general population.

Still, for years government officials have been wary of the tattoo and body-piercing industry, and for many decades several states outlawed tattooing and piercing altogether out of fear that unclean needles could help spread hepatitis. In 2006 Oklahoma became the last state to legalize tattooing. Under law in Oklahoma, as well as in many other states, tattoo artists must be licensed by the state, agree to regular inspections conducted by the state health department, and take courses in preventing blood contamination.

> The cost of living with hepatitis C does not end with the cost of the drug therapy. Hepatitis patients are often ill for months and unable to work; their families suffer because of loss of income.

Many professional tattoo artists and body piercers endorse such regulations, believing they are necessary to keep amateurs, whom they call "scratchers," out of the business. "These are guys who can't afford to sterilize their equipment and may be spreading diseases like hepatitis and AIDS," tattoo artist Darrell McWilliams told the *Oregonian* newspaper. "They do tattoos at their houses or at parties, and people assume they're safe because they know the guy or their friend knows him. It's not safe."[26]

Despite the precautions taken by government regulators and the tattoo and body-piercing industry, health professionals maintain that customers should be wary of needles. "There are a lot of risks for hepatitis C, which can be very aggressive and life threatening," Texas physician Donovan Sigerfoos told *Texas Monthly* magazine. "You need to pick a place that can verify that they use disposable products and that they're not recycling inks and needles even if they advertise that they sterilize them. Make sure it looks like a nice clean shop."[27]

Strain on Prisons

Tattooing is also a routine part of prison life in America. Modern, sanitary tattooing equipment is not available to inmates because prison officials regard it as contraband—prohibited items. Still, prison inmates want tattoos, which means amateur artists do a brisk business behind jailhouse walls. They fashion their needles out of Bic pens and similar implements and grind down the graphite in pencils, which they use as ink.

This illegal tattoo trade has led to a hepatitis epidemic in American prisons. In 2000 the U.S. Justice Department found that 31 percent of the hepatitis C tests administered in American prisons showed positive results. Critics charge that the problem may be even more widespread because corrections officials in the United States may be testing only a fraction of the nation's 2 million inmates.

> Despite the precautions taken by government regulators and the tattoo and body-piercing industry, health professionals maintain that customers should be wary of needles.

In recent years charges have surfaced accusing prison administrators of withholding hepatitis testing and treatment from inmates, hoping to have them finish their sentences before their liver damage becomes too pronounced. By discharging the inmates without treating them, critics argue, prison officials can avoid the high cost of hepatitis care. Indeed, in 2006 family members of Oregon prison inmate Rodger Anstett sued the state, claiming prison officials let the inmate die rather than treat his hepatitis. What is more, critics believe that the Justice Department's study may have actually underreported the number of hepatitis cases in American prisons because many corrections officials do no testing at all. Michelle Burrows, an attorney who represents the Anstett family in the lawsuit, told the magazine *Progressive*, "Most prison systems are purposely not testing for hep C so they can say 'we don't know who's got it,' and don't have to treat it."[28] In fact, the *Progressive* article reported that when the Anstett suit was filed, Oregon prisons held more than 3,500 inmates who had tested positive for hepatitis C, yet just a dozen prisoners received medical treatment.

Corrections officials argue that they are responsible for maintaining county and state prisons on limited budgets and that taxpayers question how lawbreakers can be given access to free medical care when many working people cannot afford to pay the high cost of doctors and prescription drugs. Joseph Bick, chief medical officer for the California Medical Prison Facility in Vacaville, California, told the Associated Press, "It's a hard sell to convince taxpayers why additional resources should be spent on the health care of the incarcerated when there are a lot of people who aren't incarcerated who don't have adequate health care."[29]

> " **Charges have surfaced accusing prison administrators of withholding hepatitis testing and treatment from inmates, hoping to have them finish their sentences before their liver damage becomes too pronounced.** "

In Oregon the Anstett lawsuit was effective in forcing the state prison system to upgrade medical care for hepatitis patients. Attorneys reached a settlement requiring the state to initiate hepatitis C tests for all prison inmates. What is more, outside medical experts were brought in to craft a treatment program for inmates who test positive for the disease. Under the settlement, Oregon can withhold treatment only for inmates whose sentences would end before they would start to show benefits from the drug therapy.

Hepatitis and the Immigration Debate

For years Congress has wrestled with the issue of how to stem the flow of illegal immigrants into the United States. Experts say that about 10 million illegal immigrants were living in the United States in 2005. Many critics believe that people entering the country illegally are already stricken with infectious diseases, particularly hepatitis. Critics also point to the fact that Latin America and Asia have some of the highest rates of hepatitis B and C in the world and suggest that even legal immigrants from those countries be monitored for hepatitis. According to the Asian Liver Center at Stanford University in California, more than half of the 1.3 million new cases of hepatitis B reported each year in the United States afflict Asians. "We hope the government will pass a bill that requires every immigrant to be tested for hepatitis B,"[30] Jordan Su, program manager at the Asian Liver Center, told the *Washington Times.*

Studies show that Hispanic immigrants suffer from higher than average infection rates for hepatitis A. Fernando Guerra, director of the San Antonio Metropolitan Health District in Texas, told *Hispanic* magazine, "Hepatitis A is related to the movement of people across the binational border. We need to make people aware of the risk."[31]

Such admissions by physicians and Hispanic leaders have fueled calls for tough anti-immigration laws by social conservatives and others who oppose immigration. Before she died in 2006, California-based attorney Madeleine Cosman, an expert in medical law, argued strongly for laws that would screen immigrants for diseases, particularly hepatitis. Appearing on CNN in 2005, Cosman said, "Certain diseases that we thought we had vanquished years ago are coming back. And other diseases that we've never seen or rarely seen in America, because they've always been the diseases of poverty and the Third World, are coming in now."[32]

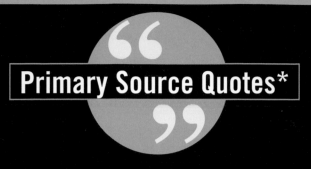

What Are the Social Impacts of Hepatitis?

66 People, in general, bring in diseases from their home countries. But I don't want to say all immigrants are carrying diseases. 99

—Walter Tsou, quoted in Joyce Howard Price, "Disease, Unwanted Import," *Washington Times*, February 13, 2005.

Tsou is president of the American Public Health Association.

66 When I tell young Chinese people they have to take a lifetime worth of drugs for a virus that is currently giving them no symptoms, they don't understand that. Then they refuse and remain carriers and can pass the virus on. 99

—Sing Chan, quoted in Corey Kilgannon, "So Many Hepatitis Cases, So Many Cures," *New York Times*, May 13, 2006.

Chan is a liver specialist practicing in New York City.

* Editor's Note: While the definition of a primary source can be narrowly or broadly defined, for the purposes of Compact Research, a primary source consists of: 1) results of original research presented by an organization or researcher; 2) eyewitness accounts of events, personal experience, or work experience; 3) first-person editorials offering pundits' opinions; 4) government officials presenting political plans and/or policies; 5) representatives of organizations presenting testimony or policy.

Primary Source Quotes

❝Due to the transmission through contaminated water and food, and high rates of international exchanges, the rate of hepatitis is likely to remain in the border region.❞

—U.S./Mexico Border Counties Coalition, *At the Crossroads: U.S. Mexico Border Counties in Transition*, March 2006. www.bordercounties.org.

The U.S./Mexico Border Counties Coalition is composed of the 24 counties in Texas, Arizona, New Mexico, and California that share a common border with Mexico; the coalition studies immigration issues and lobbies for changes in national immigration laws.

❝I actually made a syringe out of a Bic pen. If you get one set of [needle and ink], the whole wing's using it. And that's how [AIDS] and hepatitis C are spread. That's where I believe I got it.❞

—"Greg," quoted in Kai Wright, "Prison Outbreak: An Epidemic of Hepatitis C," *Progressive*, March 2006.

"Greg" is a former inmate of a New Jersey prison and amateur tattoo artist.

❝We realized that the state of Pennsylvania has no regulations for tattoo businesses, and board members saw this potential for disease.❞

—Andy Glass, quoted in David Bruce, "Parlor Protection," *Oregonian*, August 30, 2006.

Glass, director of the Erie County Department of Health, explains why Erie County, Pennsylvania, officials enacted a local ordinance requiring health inspections of tattoo parlors.

❝There is no reason for every 25-year-old woman with a butterfly on her shoulder to get tested. But people thinking of having their bodies pierced or tattooed should look for the highest standard of infection control. Anything that pierces your skin can transmit a blood-borne infection.❞

—Miriam Alter, quoted in Geoffrey Cowley et al., "Hepatitis C: The Insidious Spread of a Killer Virus," *Newsweek*, April 22, 2002.

Alter is an epidemiologist for the U.S. Centers for Disease Control and Prevention.

❝They give us a big speech to not get tattoos in here.❞

—Sean Barnett, quoted in Cheryl Corley, "North Dakota Takes on Hepatitis C in Prisons," *Morning Edition*, National Public Radio, June 6, 2007.

Barnett is an inmate at a state prison in Bismarck, North Dakota.

....

❝Injection of drugs is far and away the number one way [hepatitis] transmits. And then also here culturally when folks are in prison, there's a lot of body art, a lot of tattooing, a lot of body piercing. And it really is a way to express yourself in a place where you can't express yourself.❞

—John Hagen, quoted in Cheryl Corley, "North Dakota Takes on Hepatitis C in Prisons," *Morning Edition*, National Public Radio, June 6, 2007.

Hagen is a staff physician for the North Dakota state prison system.

....

❝Even though most immigrants come from countries poorer than the United States, recent immigrants are healthier than the U.S.-born population in virtually every particular.❞

—Southern Poverty Law Center, "The Immigrants: Myths and Realities," *Southern Poverty Law Center Intelligence Report 2001*. www.splcenter.org.

The Southern Poverty Law Center reports on the activities of hate groups and provides legal assistance to clients who oppose discriminatory practices by governments, individuals, and groups.

....

❝They gave me shots for hep A and B, got rid of them. I'd like to get rid of the C, too. I'm entitled to that. But some docs will give you the treatment and others won't. I keep making appointments. I keep asking.❞

—Anthony Harris, quoted in Martha Mendoza, "Prisons Breed Hepatitis C Victims; Nobody Knows How Many Inmates Have the Disease, Which Can Be Treated," *Pittsburgh Post-Gazette*, Associated Press, March 18, 2007.

Harris is an inmate serving a life sentence in a California prison.

....

What Are the Social Impacts of Hepatitis?

- Depression may influence how quickly hepatitis patients recover from their illness. A 2005 study conducted by Emory University in Georgia showed that **34 percent** of patients suffering severe depression recovered from hepatitis within 24 weeks, while **60 percent** of patients with mild depression cleared the virus from their systems much faster.

- **Massachusetts legalized tattooing in 2000**. The art had been banned in the state since 1962 after a hepatitis outbreak in New York state was linked to tattoo artists.

- Many Asian hepatitis victims living in the United States who cannot afford expensive drugs turn to **herbal medicines** such as lotus seeds, ginseng root, ginkgo, shark cartilage, and fish oil. Doctors insist those remedies will not cure liver disease.

- Prison tattoo artists are known to **steal used hypodermic needles** from waste baskets in the jail infirmaries; they smuggle them back to their cells and fashion them into tattoo needles.

- Autoimmune hepatitis is rare, affecting fewer than **200 victims for every 1 million people**.

- Physicians believe that **6 percent** of mothers afflicted with hepatitis C pass the disease on to their babies.

Hepatitis by Gender

Studies show that women who contract hepatitis are more likely to suffer from depression than are men, but men are more likely to contract the disease. Public health researchers believe men are more likely than women to engage in the type of risky behavior that leads to hepatitis infections. Statistics compiled by the U.S. Centers for Disease Control and Prevention show that in 2005, more men than women contracted the acute infections of hepatitis A, B, and C. The CDC does not compile statistics by gender on the chronic infections of hepatitis B and C; nevertheless, since all hepatitis cases begin as acute infections, these statistics provide evidence that men are more likely than women to contract hepatitis in any of its forms.

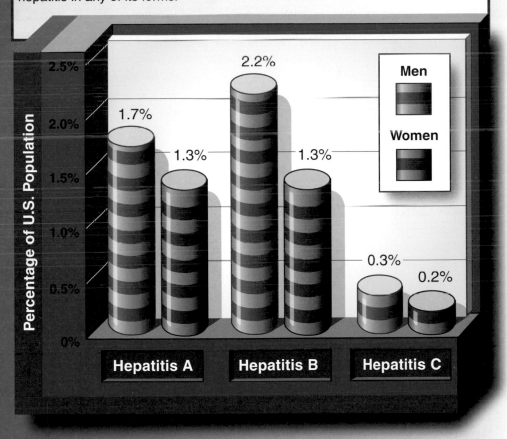

Source: U.S. Centers for Disease Control and Prevention, "Summary of Notifiable Diseases, 2005," *Morbidity and Mortality Weekly Report*, March 30, 2007. www.cdc.gov.

Hepatitis A Cases Among Hispanics and Non-Hispanics

Hispanic immigrants are suspected of spreading hepatitis in the United States. Statistics compiled by the U.S. Centers for Disease Control and Prevention indicate that the infection rate for hepatitis A among Hispanics is far greater than for people of non-Hispanic ethnicity. In 2005, in cases in which ethnicity is known, more than 1,100 new cases of hepatitis A were reported among Hispanics in America, while non-Hispanics reported about 2,000 new cases. Therefore, more than 33 percent of the new cases of hepatitis A were reported among Hispanics, even though they make up just 14 percent of the U.S. population. Since hepatitis A is spread through fecal contamination of food and water, a large measure of the infections may stem from the unsanitary conditions in which illegal immigrants are forced to live, particularly in the border states of Texas, Arizona, New Mexico, and California.

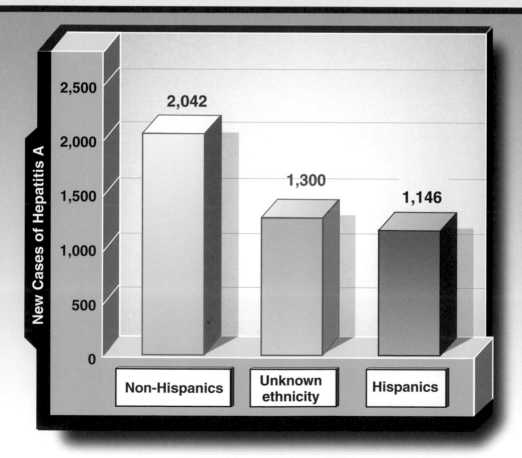

Source: U.S. Centers for Disease Control and Prevention, "Summary of Notifiable Diseases, 2005," *Morbidity and Mortality Weekly Report,* March 30, 2007. www.cdc.gov.

Hepatitis B and C in American Prisons

In 2001, nearly 2 million Americans were incarcerated in prisons, where many of them contracted hepatitis B and C. According to the U.S. Centers for Disease Control and Prevention, between 1 and 3.7 percent of the American prison population has contracted hepatitis B, while between 12 and 35 percent of inmates may suffer from hepatitis C. Among the reasons for the high rates of the 2 diseases: Amateur tattoo artists who use dirty needles, intravenous drug abuse behind bars, and sex among inmates.

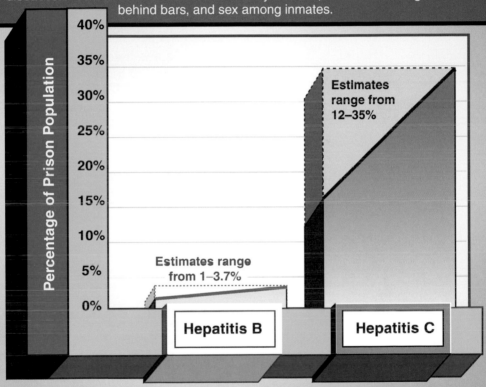

Source: Cindy Weinbaum, Rob Lyerla, and Harold S. Margolis, U.S. Centers for Disease Control and Prevention, Division of Viral Hepatitis, "Prevention and Control of Infections with Hepatitis Viruses in Correctional Settings," *Morbidity and Mortality Weekly Report*, January 24, 2003. www.cdc.gov.

- According to the U.S. Centers for Disease Control and Prevention, more than **150,000 former prison inmates** suffer from hepatitis B, while more than 1.3 million former inmates suffer from hepatitis C.

- According to the U.S. Centers for Disease Control and Prevention, as many as **6 percent** of juveniles held in detention centers are afflicted with hepatitis B.

Hepatitis and the Asian Community

New York University found that hepatitis B afflicts a high percentage of the Asian community in New York City, which totals about 800,000 people. According to the study, between 12.5 and 17 percent of the Asians living in New York are afflicted with the disease. Many of the victims have lived in the United States for less than 5 years, which has fueled charges that Asian immigrants are bringing the disease into America. Many of the infected Asians have immigrated to the United States from China and South Korea.

Hepatitis B infections among Asians living in New York City in 2005 by country of birth

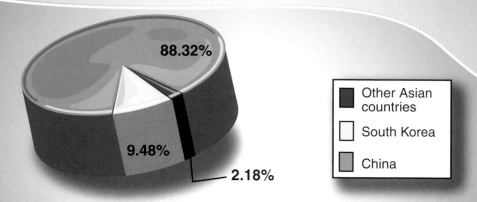

88.32%

9.48%

2.18%

- Other Asian countries
- South Korea
- China

Hepatitis B infections among Asians living in New York City in 2005 by years in the United States

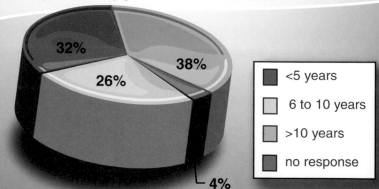

32%

38%

26%

4%

- <5 years
- 6 to 10 years
- >10 years
- no response

Source: U.S. Centers for Disease Control and Prevention, "Screening for Chronic Hepatitis B Among Asian/Pacific Islander Populations–New York City, 2005," *Morbidity and Mortality Weekly Report*, May 12, 2006. www.cdc.gov.

- All survivors of terrorist attacks in Israel are **vaccinated for hepatitis B**. The Israeli government instituted the policy after blood samples taken from the remains of two suicide bombers in 2001 indicated the terrorists had the disease.

- In Texas communities along the Mexican border, about **400,000 illegal immigrants** do not have access to clean water or sewer systems, making them prime candidates for hepatitis A, according to reports compiled by the U.S.-Mexico Border Counties Coalition and the Federal Reserve Bank of Dallas.

- Although far less common than tattooing, acupuncture has occasionally been identified as the cause of hepatitis. **Acupuncture** is an ancient healing practice in which needles are inserted into energy pathways to relieve pain. For example, in 1984, 35 patients of a Rhode Island acupuncturist contracted hepatitis B during their treatments.

- **Tongue and genital piercing** can spread hepatitis B and C during sex, even if a condom is worn. Public health officials suggest that condoms can be torn by tongue and genital jewelry, thereby breaking down the protection provided by the condom.

- A 2004 study by Duke University found that antiviral drugs work just **19 percent** of the time in African American patients. This is in contrast to a **50 percent** overall success rate in non–African American hepatitis B or C patients.

Can Hepatitis Be Prevented?

> **66** By a strange irony, the blood of people who had already been exposed to the virus and developed an antibody against it could be used to detect the virus present in donors' blood and prevent its use to infect others. **99**

> —Baruch S. Blumberg, winner of the Nobel Prize in Physiology or Medicine for research that led to the hepatitis B vaccine.

Hepatitis remains a significant public health concern in the United States, but unquestionably, far fewer people suffer from the affliction now than ever before. After reaching a peak in the early 1960s when hepatitis A afflicted more than 40 out of every 100,000 people, the spread of the disease has declined to fewer than 2 out of every 100,000 people. The rates of hepatitis B and C have declined as well, due mostly to improved public education about the diseases, better monitoring of donated blood, and the widespread use of the hepatitis B vaccine, which is administered to most school-age children in America. What is more, due to the diligence of public health authorities, occurrences of hepatitis D and E remain rare in the United States.

Annemarie Wasley, an epidemiologist at the U.S. Centers for Disease Control and Prevention, told the *New York Times*, "We're doing a good job at preventing new cases, but we still have a large burden of chronic B and C, and we have to reach out to these people to prevent transmission to others and to help them maintain their own health."[33]

Success on a global scale has been mixed. Since 1991 the World Health Organization has called on nations to administer the hepatitis

B vaccine to their citizens. Nearly 120 countries have agreed to add the vaccine to their national immunization programs, but many developing countries in Africa, Asia, and elsewhere that cannot afford expensive drugs have been unable to establish widespread inoculation programs. As a result, even though a vaccine for hepatitis B has been available since 1986, the disease remains a worldwide danger to public health, causing more than 1 million deaths a year.

The Australia Antigen

Nevertheless, in countries in which the hepatitis B vaccine is available, it is likely that the immunization has saved millions of lives. Indeed, discovery of the hepatitis B vaccine is regarded as one of the most important accomplishments in the history of medicine. In 1976 the Nobel Prize for Physiology or Medicine was awarded to biochemist Baruch S. Blumberg, whose research led to the development of the hepatitis B vaccine.

Blumberg had not been searching for a vaccine for hepatitis B. Instead, he was studying blood proteins—chemicals that determine different blood types such as A and O. Blumberg theorized that people who receive many blood transfusions, such as hemophiliacs, develop immune reactions, or antibodies, that help them absorb the foreign proteins, or antigens, in the blood they receive from others. Blumberg traveled the world collecting blood samples. In 1963 he found that blood from a hemophilia patient from New York City had developed antibodies to an antigen that was present in the blood of an Australian aborigine.

At this point, Blumberg knew there was something wrong with the aborigine's blood, but he did not know that it was hepatitis. For the next three years Blumberg and other members of his research team tested the blood of others, looking for the cause of the antigen. They concentrated on patients with the bone marrow cancer known as leukemia as well as children with Down

> " Even though a vaccine for hepatitis B has been available since 1986, the disease remains a worldwide danger to public health, causing more than 1 million deaths a year. "

syndrome, a cause of mental retardation. In 1966 they found the Australia antigen in the blood of a 12-year-old boy with Down syndrome who also suffered from hepatitis B. That led them to make further tests on hepatitis B patients, whose blood also contained the Australia antigen. Now, it was clear that the Australia antigen was a virus—hepatitis B.

The first outcome of Blumberg's research was the development of a test for the Australia antigen. Another Nobel Prize–winning scientist, Rosalyn Yalow, had developed a method for detecting how viruses react to antibodies. Yalow's method was applied to the Australia antigen. The process proved to be an accurate method for testing blood for hepatitis B. In 1972 Congress mandated that all donated blood used for transfusions be tested for hepatitis B. Also, hepatitis B screening has become a routine test administered to all pregnant women in the United States.

> **It was clear the Australia antigen was a virus—hepatitis B.**

It took several more years of research and development, but eventually a vaccine for hepatitis B was developed. Blumberg and other researchers determined that some patients develop a natural immunity to the disease. They believed the antibodies of people who were naturally immune to the disease could be used to produce a vaccine. Private drug companies, which were already investing heavily in developing a vaccine for the disease, announced a breakthrough in 1981, when they produced a vaccine made from the blood of patients infected with hepatitis B. It took another five years of research and development before the U.S. Food and Drug Administration (FDA) approved the distribution of the vaccine. Perhaps the most significant achievement of the hepatitis B vaccine is that it is one of the few immunizations that can prevent cancer. Since hepatitis B can ultimately result in cancer of the liver, somebody vaccinated against the disease will be protected against one of the major causes of liver cancer.

Hepatitis C: No Protection

In 1995 a vaccine was produced for the hepatitis A virus by competing research teams at two major American drug companies, Merck & Co.,

Inc. and SmithKline Beecham. The biochemists who developed the vaccines were able to isolate the hepatitis A virus in a culture dish and then kill it with a toxic chemical known as formalin, which is similar to formaldehyde, the substance used to preserve lab specimens.

Since hepatitis A is contracted as an acute disease only and is generally not regarded as life-threatening, governments have in the past not mandated widespread immunization programs. For years the hepatitis A vaccine has been administered only to children in high-risk areas, usually in rural regions of the United States with large populations of American Indians and Native Alaskans. Others who are urged to get the vaccine are people who travel to countries where the purity of the food and water is suspect, health care and day care workers, gay men with multiple partners, and others whose activities place them at a high risk to contract the disease. However, since the hepatitis A vaccine has been found to be particularly effective—the immunizations have reduced the number of cases in the United States from 143,000 in 2000 to 61,000 in 2003—in 2005 the CDC urged all states to adopt mandatory hepatitis A vaccination programs for all children between 12 and 23 months old. Harold Margolis, the former director of viral hepatitis research at the CDC, told *Hispanic* magazine, "The strategy for controlling hepatitis A is similar to the one we are using to control polio: widespread catch-up immunization of young, susceptible children followed by routine immunization."[34]

No vaccines have yet been developed for hepatitis C, D, and E. Although major pharmaceutical companies in the United States and other countries have made major investments in searching for a cure for hepatitis C, the vaccine remains elusive. Also, given the limited effectiveness of interferon and ribavirin, many drug companies have invested in new treatments for people already infected with hepatitis C and the other forms of the disease. Again, though, no new effective treatments have

> " Although major pharmaceutical companies in the United States and other countries have made major investments in searching for a cure for hepatitis C, the vaccine remains elusive. "

been developed. States *Economist* magazine, "In practice, it is unlikely that any one medication will be enough to beat hepatitis C. Just as with [AIDS]—and, indeed, the existing interferon-ribavirin approach—a combination of drugs, attacking the problem from different angles, will probably be the most potent weapon."[35]

Research Continues

Science is also exploring other ways to help hepatitis patients recover. For example, medical researchers are pursuing the transplantation of not just whole or partial livers, but of liver cells. In laboratory tests on mice, healthy liver cells have been injected into diseased livers, where they have regenerated and grown into healthy liver tissue. Some experiments have seen new cells create new liver tissue that has grown to as much as 30 percent of the mass of a normal mouse liver. "That is enough liver mass to insure survival of the individual when it is combined with the original liver," says physician and author James L. Achord. "If this procedure can be reproduced in human subjects, it holds a great deal of promise. . . . For those with chronic liver disease who are not candidates for whole organ transplants, it could be life saving."[36]

> Despite loud protests from gay rights leaders, the FDA has steadfastly refused to alter a long-standing policy that prohibits gay men from donating blood.

Achord also believes that embryonic stem cell research may hold great promise for people with diseased livers. Stem cells are withdrawn from the human embryos that have been created not through the human sexual act but at in vitro fertilization clinics, where the egg is withdrawn from the mother and fertilized outside the womb. Since just one embryo is returned to the mother's womb at the clinic, the others are discarded but frequently donated by the couples to laboratories that pursue stem cell research.

It is believed that embryonic stem cells can be cultured to create all manner of human cells and that stem cells hold great promise for eradicating disease by replacing diseased cells with healthy cells. Some researchers believe they can be used to grow new organs, including the liver. "Current research in manipulating stem cells to grow new livers holds tremendous potential for replacement of diseased livers," says Achord.[37]

However, embryonic stem cell research has faced stiff political opposition in the United States. Conservative politicians oppose the research, arguing that embryos—even those that are just a few days old—are human lives, and that they should not be destroyed under any circumstances, even in the pursuit of medical research that could

> " Programs to provide immunizations are often thwarted by corrupt strongmen who are suspicious of Western-sponsored humanitarian aid. "

save others. For years, the U.S. government has cut off most funding for embryonic stem cell research programs, but state governments and private donors have made up some of the lost funding. Clearly, the debate in Washington over stem cell research will continue for years.

Refining Rules and Laws

In the United States public health officials as well as legislators and public advocacy groups are constantly reviewing research and refining rules and laws that help guard against the spread of hepatitis. For example, in 2006 the CDC launched a major study that is intended to once and for all settle the question of whether people who undergo tattooing and body piercing are at a high risk for contracting hepatitis B and C.

Some communities do not plan to wait for the outcome of the CDC study. In 2007 officials of Suffolk County, a suburban area of New York City, proposed a ban on several types of tattoos and body piercings in an effort to control the spread of infections, including hepatitis. According to estimates, the 45 tattoo parlors in Suffolk County perform some 100,000 tattoos and piercings a year. Public health officials believe that such a high number of tattoos and piercings will inevitably lead to the spread of disease. By late 2007 Suffolk County officials had not yet acted on the proposal. After tattoo shop owners protested the pending ban, county officials agreed to set up a committee that includes tattoo artists and physicians to study proposed changes in the county's health code.

Meanwhile, despite loud protests from gay rights leaders, the FDA has steadfastly refused to alter a long-standing policy that prohibits gay men from donating blood. The policy was enacted in 1985 as the AIDS epidemic spread throughout the gay community. FDA officials believe the ban on donations by gay men ensures the nation's blood supply will remain free of infection from other diseases as well, including hepatitis. But with effective tests to screen hepatitis carriers, gay activists insist the ban discriminates against them.

Gay rights leaders have been joined in their cause by officials from the American Red Cross, which collects 45 percent of all blood donated in the United States. The Red Cross, which occasionally finds itself in short supply of blood that it provides to hospitals, believes that gay men should have the right to participate in the organization's blood drives. In 2006 the Red Cross issued a statement calling the ban on donations by gay men "unfair and discriminatory," adding, "It does not appear rational to treat gay sex differently from straight sex."[38] Still, the FDA has maintained its ban.

International Efforts

Efforts to prevent hepatitis elsewhere in the world are often based on the cooperation of the governments in countries where the disease presents a threat to public health. Indeed, some of the world's poorest nations are led by some of the world's cruelest dictators. As such, programs to provide immunizations are often thwarted by corrupt strongmen who are suspicious of Western-sponsored humanitarian aid. Unquestionably, hepatitis runs rampant in Sudan, where President Omar al-Bashir, in power since 1989, has waged war against the country's non-Islamic citizens, driving some 2 million people from their homes in Darfur into unsanitary and disease-ridden refugee camps.

Elsewhere, the despotic regime of President Islam Karimov in Uzbekistan has prevented Western aid from reaching his beleaguered people. As a result, nearly 1 in 10 Uzbeks are afflicted with hepatitis B. According to the National Institutes of Health, more than 3,000 Uzbeks die each year of liver disease that is directly attributable to the virus.

Still, some immunization campaigns do reach needy people. Many of those campaigns are conducted by the GAVI Alliance, which was formerly known as the Global Alliance for Vaccines and Immunization. The alliance is a consortium of international governments and private foundations based in Geneva, Switzerland. Since its establishment in 2000, GAVI Alliance has provided hepatitis B immunizations to 126 million children. It has also distributed more than 1.2 billion disposable syringes to health care workers in dozens of developing nations to assure that hepatitis and other blood-borne diseases are not passed on accidentally.

Among the countries that have accepted aid from GAVI Alliance is China, which for decades maintained a closed society in an effort to keep out Western influences. In recent years, though, China has invited warmer relations with the West. As a result, the country has taken steps to immunize its citizens. Starting in 2002 China accepted aid from GAVI Alliance to provide hepatitis B vaccines; since then, more than 11 million Chinese children have received immunizations against the disease. Said Gao Qiang, minister of health in China, "Our goal is to protect all the babies at birth from this virus."[39]

Prognosis for the Future

The effort by China shows that with cooperation of the government, it is possible to greatly reduce the spread of hepatitis B. Hepatitis A can also be controlled through vaccinations. Sadly, not all governments are willing to cooperate, and that is why hepatitis A and B remain public health concerns even though science has shown that the diseases can be eradicated. As for hepatitis C and the other forms of the disease, medical researchers acknowledge that they are perhaps years away from developing effective vaccines as well as treatments that will show higher rates of success than interferon and ribavirin. Until then, the best way for people to prevent the spread of hepatitis is to avoid the risks by staying away from drugs, practicing safe sex, and maintaining a clean and healthy lifestyle.

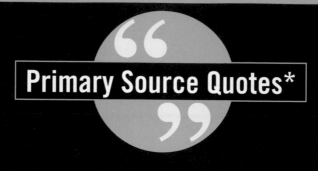

Primary Source Quotes*

Can Hepatitis Be Prevented?

66 We now have evidence that it is possible to rapidly scale up access to vaccines and that even poor countries with few resources can obtain brilliant outcomes if given the opportunity. 99

—Julian Lob-Levyt, quoted in GAVI Alliance, "Dramatic Progress in GAVI's First Five Years Shapes Next Steps in Plan to Boost Vaccinations, Save Millions of World's Poor Children," news release, December 9, 2005. www.gavialliance.org.

Lob-Levyt is executive secretary of GAVI Alliance.

66 The holy grail of hep C treatment will be if you can give therapy for 12 weeks max, with drugs that are less toxic. 99

—Greg Dore, quoted in Adam Cresswell, "The Hidden Epidemic," *Australian* (Sydney), September 30, 2006.

Dore is head of the viral hepatitis clinical research program at the University of New South Wales, Australia.

* Editor's Note: While the definition of a primary source can be narrowly or broadly defined, for the purposes of Compact Research, a primary source consists of: 1) results of original research presented by an organization or researcher; 2) eyewitness accounts of events, personal experience, or work experience; 3) first-person editorials offering pundits' opinions; 4) government officials presenting political plans and/or policies; 5) representatives of organizations presenting testimony or policy.

66 There's been a flurry of research activity. . . . We've gone from treatments that are less than 10 percent effective to therapies now that are 50 percent effective. We feel that if we can eradicate the virus, we call that a cure. 99

—Fred Poordad, quoted in Anita Manning, "Hepatitis, 'the Silent Killer,' Driven Out of the Shadows; New Medications, Research Bring Hope, Treatment, Even Cures," *USA Today*, January 23, 2006.

Poordad is chief of hepatology at the Center for Liver Disease and Transplantation at Cedars-Sinai Medical Center, Los Angeles, California.

66 All men who seek to donate blood are asked if they have had sex, even once, with another man since 1977. Those who say they have are permanently banned from donating blood. 99

News Rx, *Medical Letter on the CDC & FDA*, September 25, 2000.

News Rx is a service that provides news items culled from 5,000 medical publications to subscribers.

66 Hepatitis B represents a huge health problem in Uzbekistan, especially in young adults. The potential for prevention by vaccination seems very high, but demands a long-term vision if chronic hepatitis, in particular, is to be reduced. 99

—P. Beutels, E.I. Musabaev, Philip Van Damme, and T. Yasin, "The Disease Burden of Hepatitis B in Uzbekistan," *Journal of Infection*, October 2000.

Beutels, Musabaev, Van Damme, and Yasin are affiliated with the Department of Epidemiology and Community Medicine, University of Antwerp, Belgium.

66 The most significant outcome of our research has, probably, been the invention and the introduction of the hepatitis B vaccine, one of the most widely used vaccines in the world and the first 'cancer vaccine.' **99**

—Baruch S. Blumberg, *Hepatitis B: The Hunt for a Killer Virus.* Princeton, NJ: Princeton University Press, 2002.

Blumberg won the Nobel Prize in Physiology or Medicine for the research that led to development of the hepatitis B vaccine.

66 The hepatitis B vaccine is very safe. Minor reactions to it may occur in a small number of children and can include fussiness as well as redness, soreness, or swelling where the shot is given. A mild fever may occur as well. **99**

—Margaret C. Fisher, ed., *Immunizations & Infectious Diseases.* Elk Grove Village, IL: American Academy of Pediatrics, 2006.

Fisher is professor of pediatrics at the Drexel University College of Medicine, Philadelphia, Pennsylvania.

66 A good source of liver cells would be beneficial to many, many people. If we could get a liver cell line that was immortal—one that could divide and grow indefinitely—then we could give new liver cells to anyone who needs them. **99**

—Mark Zern, quoted in UC Davis Health System, "Mark Zern: Meeting Challenges, Leading the Way." www.ucdmc.ucdavis.edu.

Zern is the director of the transplant research program at the University of California at Davis School of Medicine.

66 Our treatments of both acute and chronic hepatitis leave much to be desired, but current research promises better results in the future. **99**

—James L. Achord, *Understanding Hepatitis.* Jackson: University Press of Mississippi, 2002.

Achord is professor emeritus at the University of Mississippi Medical Center and has written extensively on liver disease.

66A newborn who becomes infected with hepatitis B has a 90 percent chance of becoming chronically infected with the virus. . . . Thus, if you are pregnant, you should be screened for hepatitis B.99

—Sanjiv Chopra, *Dr. Sanjiv Chopra's Liver Book*. New York: Pocket Books, 2001.

Chopra is a liver specialist and associate professor of medicine at Harvard Medical School in Massachusetts.

66Starting with children, the vaccine project is a step forward to help the nation finally shake off its notoriety as the major hepatitis B host.99

—Wang Zhao, quoted in Shan Juan, "China Has 120 Million Hepatitis B Carriers," *China Daily*, September 1, 2007.

Wang is vice president of the China Foundation for Hepatitis Prevention and Control.

66The hepatitis B vaccine represents one of the most important advances in the medical field. This is the first and only vaccine in history that can simultaneously prevent liver cancer, cirrhosis, and a sexually transmitted disease—hepatitis B.99

—Melissa Palmer, *Melissa Palmer's Guide to Hepatitis Liver Disease*. Garden City Park, NY: Avery, 2000.

Palmer is a liver specialist who practices in New York.

Facts and Illustrations

Can Hepatitis Be Prevented?

- Prior to the development of the **hepatitis B screening test**, 50 percent of all patients who received blood transfusions for major surgeries contracted the disease.

- According to the U.S. Centers for Disease Control and Prevention, since 1986 less than **1 percent** of people with tattoos contracted hepatitis C. The CDC believes, however, that those statistics do not tell the true story of whether tattoo needles spread hepatitis, and it has initiated a thorough study of the issue.

- Drug maker Hoffman-LaRoche Inc., which manufactures an interferon-based hepatitis treatment marketed under the name Pegasys, sold **$1.4 billion** worth of the drug to hepatitis C patients in 2005.

- In 2005 the World Bank, which helps fund international immunization programs, reported that as many as **70 percent of the 4 billion vaccinations** administered in India were either improperly administered or performed with needles that were not sterilized.

- The original hepatitis B vaccine was made from the blood of people who developed antibodies to the virus; in the late 1980s a synthetic version was developed, and **now most people are immunized** with the updated vaccine, which is known as Recombivax. Blood is no longer employed as the vaccine's main component; it has been replaced by baker's yeast.

Sexually Transmitted Diseases Among Pregnant Women

Although infection of newborns by their mothers is rare, the U.S. Centers for Disease Control and Prevention urges all pregnant women to be tested for hepatitis B and C. According to statistics compiled by the CDC, hepatitis B is one of the most common sexually transmitted diseases that afflicts pregnant women. If a mother-to-be tests positive for hepatitis B, doctors can administer a vaccine to the baby within 12 hours of delivery. If a baby contracts hepatitis B by ingesting the mother's blood during delivery and is not vaccinated, studies show that 90 percent of infected babies will develop hepatitis B and suffer liver damage later in life.

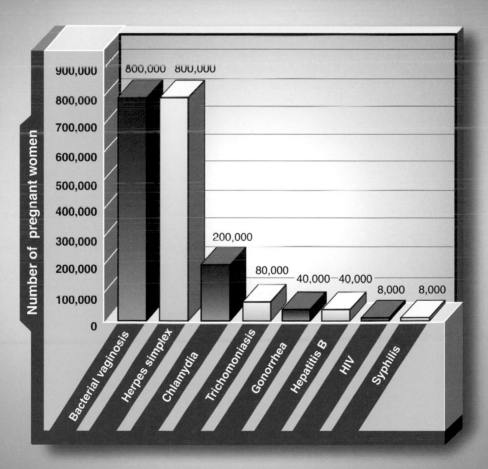

Source: "STDs and Pregnancy–CDC Fact Sheet," www.cdc.gov.

Hepatitis Vaccinations

Two decades after the hepatitis B vaccine was developed, most states
kindergarten. Six states that do not require the immunization are
(Vermont and South Dakota recommend that parents have their children
urged all states to require immunizations against hepatitis A for all
vaccines before entering kindergarten. They are Alaska, Texas,

2005–2006 Hepatitis B Vaccination Requirements by State (for Kindergarten)

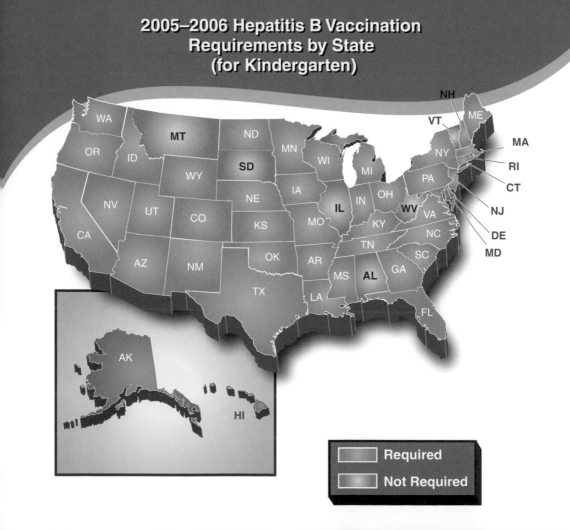

Required
Not Required

require all school children to receive the immunization before starting
Montana, Alabama, Illinois, West Virginia, Vermont, and South Dakota
immunized). The U.S. Centers for Disease Control and Prevention
young children. As of 2006, six states require children to receive the
Oklahoma, Nevada, Utah, and Wyoming.

2005–2006 Hepatitis A Vaccination Requirements by State (for Kindergarten)

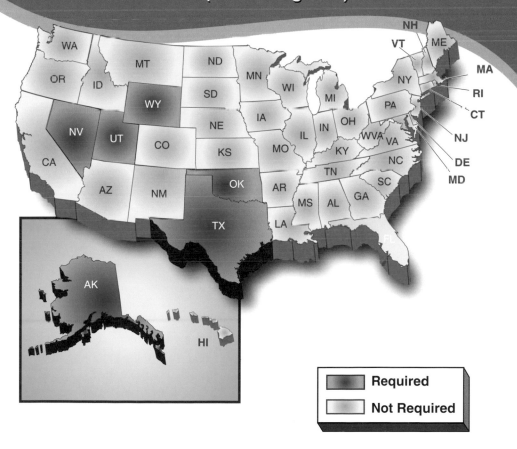

Required

Not Required

Vaccines Help Reduce Prevalence of Hepatitis A

Soon after the vaccine for hepatitis A was developed in 1995, the number of cases declined dramatically. Since hepatitis A is generally not considered to be a life-threatening disease, few state and local governments in the United States mandated its use. According to 2001 statistics, though, more than 10,000 people contracted a disease for which there is a vaccine. The vaccine has proven to be so effective, that in 2005 the U.S. Centers for Disease Control and Prevention urged state governments to mandate hepatitis A immunizations for all babies between 12 and 23 months old.

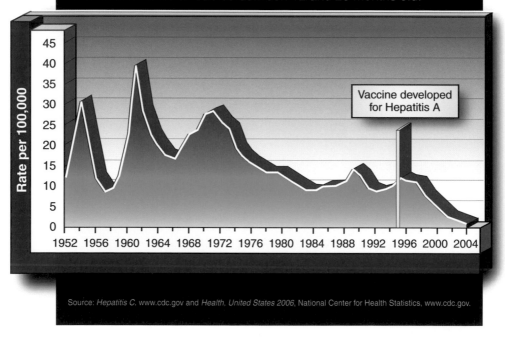

Source: *Hepatitis C*, www.cdc.gov and *Health, United States 2006*, National Center for Health Statistics, www.cdc.gov.

- Researchers at Oregon Health and Science University have successfully grown human liver cells in laboratory mice. The technique could prove to be enormously important in the **development of hepatitis drugs**, since they may now be tested on mice before undergoing human trials.

- Between **20 and 50 percent** of people who contract hepatitis C recover on their own without the need to take antiviral drugs, according to researchers at Georg-August University in Germany.

- Liver disease takes the lives of about **500,000 citizens of China** each year.

- Hepatitis E, historically confined to Asia and Africa, has started showing up in Europe. Hepatitis E can be spread from animals to people. Researchers believe the outbreak in Europe stems from **pork products infected with hepatitis E.**

- To protest against the U.S. Food and Drug Administration's ban on blood donations by gay men, hundreds of gay rights activists, mostly college students, participated in the **"Fight to Give Life" on April 5**, 2006. The activists showed up on that day at blood donation centers, offered to give blood, and acknowledged they were gay. All were turned away.

- **The livers of pigs** have occasionally been transplanted into humans as brief stopgap measures until human livers can be provided to transplant patients. Using the science of genetics, researchers believe they can eventually clone pigs with livers that could be used permanently by human liver disease sufferers.

Key People and Advocacy Groups

American Red Cross: The American Red Cross collects 45 percent of all blood donated in the United States. In 2006 the organization announced its opposition to the long-standing U.S. Food and Drug Administration ban on blood donations from gay men. The organization, as well as gay rights activists, contend that since blood can be screened for hepatitis as well as other diseases, including the virus that causes AIDS, there is no reason to continue a prohibition against blood donations from gays.

Biotechnology Industry Organization: Known as BIO, the Washington, D.C.–based group represents more than 500 American companies performing health-related research and development, including dozens that are exploring embryonic stem cell research. The trade organization lobbies members of Congress and other governmental bodies for legislation that helps enhance biotechnology research in the United States.

Baruch S. Blumberg: A biochemist, Blumberg discovered a hemophilia patient in New York who had developed antibodies to an antigen found in the blood of an aborigine in Australia. Soon, Blumberg determined the antigen was the hepatitis B virus. For that discovery, as well as his further research into how antibodies in the blood of hepatitis B patients can be used to block the virus, Blumberg was awarded the Nobel Prize.

Coalition of Americans for Research Ethics: The Washington, D.C.–based coalition opposes embryonic stem cell research, contending that embryos are human lives and should not be destroyed. Officials from the organization produce position papers and opinion pieces for newspapers and testify before Congress. Also, the coalition provides financial assistance for genetic research that does not employ embryonic stem cells, including adult stem cell research, which employs cells drawn from living adult donors.

Maurice Hilleman: Hilleman headed the research team at Merck & Co., Inc. that developed a vaccine for hepatitis A. Before he died in 2005, Hilleman helped develop a number of vaccines, including the hepatitis B vaccine as well as immunizations for measles, mumps, chickenpox, meningitis, and pneumonia.

Michael Houghton, Qui-Lim Choo, and George Kuo: Houghton, Choo, and Kuo, biochemists at Chiron Corporation, were first to identify the hepatitis C virus. They studied the genetic makeup of the virus in order to differentiate it from other forms of hepatitis. Until their breakthrough, the virus was known as "non-A, non-B" hepatitis. Victims of the virus showed all the signs of liver disease, but their bodies lacked the hepatitis A and B viruses. Once hepatitis C was identified, scientists were able to develop a test to screen donated blood for the virus. With development of the test, the number of hepatitis C cases has dropped from about 240,000 cases a year to about 26,000 cases a year.

Naomi Judd: Before Judd established a career as one of the top country-and-western singers in America, she worked as a nurse. Judd believes that at some point in the 1980s she was accidentally poked with a used intravenous needle, causing her to contract hepatitis C. Diagnosed with the disease in 1990, Judd defied her doctors' expectations that she would soon die from liver disease. She recovered and has become the public face of the disease and a dedicated spokesperson on behalf of hepatitis C research.

Latino Organization for Liver Awareness (LOLA): Founded by liver transplant patient Debbie Delgado-Vega, the New York City–based organization helps inform Hispanics of the dangers of liver disease and urges them to obtain immunizations and avoid high-risk behavior. LOLA has also developed a prison outreach project targeted at Hispanic inmates. The project advises Hispanic inmates of treatment options for hepatitis, making information available to them in Spanish.

F.O. MacCallum: During World War II, MacCallum, a British physician, observed that Allied servicemen contracted hepatitis. After further research MacCallum determined that the victims were being injected with unclean needles. In 1947 MacCallum classified the disease into hepatitis A, which he found was spread through food and water contaminated with fecal matter, and hepatitis B, which is spread through contact with contaminated blood.

National HCV Prison Coalition: Based in Eugene, Oregon, the coalition raises awareness about hepatitis C in prisons and represents inmates who have contracted the disease. In addition, the organization provides support groups for incarcerated hepatitis C patients and lobbies lawmakers to provide better hepatitis treatment programs for inmates.

U.S.-Mexico Border Counties Coalition: Composed of the 24 counties in Texas, New Mexico, Arizona, and California that border Mexico, the organization has become a leader in calling for a revision of U.S. immigration laws. The coalition's 2006 report *At the Crossroads: U.S./ Mexico Border Counties in Transition* provides statistics showing a high rate of hepatitis in communities located near the Mexican border.

Chronology

ca. 2500 B.C.
Greek physician Hippocrates first notes the symptoms of hepatitis in a patient, describing jaundice, high fever, and discolored urine.

1800s
Physicians chronicle several epidemics of jaundice, particularly in military camps where sanitation is poor and bloody wounds are common.

1962
Outbreak of hepatitis B in New York State is linked to unclean needles used by tattoo artists.

1963
Baruch S. Blumberg determines that a hemophilia patient in New York has developed antibodies to an antigen found in the blood of an aborigine in Australia.

2500 B.C.   1900   1950   1960   1970

1906
Congress adopts the U.S. Pure Food and Drug Act, establishing strict rules for sanitation in the production, shipping, and storage of food. The law helps reduce the spread of hepatitis A in the American food supply.

1955
After the Yamuna River floods in India, some 30,000 people contract hepatitis. The form of the disease they contracted is later identified as hepatitis E.

1966
Blumberg identifies the Australia antigen as hepatitis B; the discovery leads to a test for hepatitis B and development of a vaccine for the virus.

Eighth century A.D.
Pope Zacharias suggests jaundice is infectious and urges people who show the symptom to be isolated from others.

1947
British physician F.O. MacCallum determines that two types of viruses cause hepatitis, with hepatitis A spread by food and water contaminated with fecal matter, and hepatitis B spread by contaminated blood.

1972
Congress mandates all donated blood used for transfusions in the United States be tested for hepatitis B.

Chronology

1976
Blumberg is awarded Nobel Prize for the research that led to the hepatitis B vaccine.

1990
Test developed to screen donated blood for hepatitis C.

2005
U.S. Centers for Disease Control and Prevention urges all states to adopt mandatory hepatitis A immunizations for children entering kindergarten.

1986
Hepatitis B vaccine goes into widespread use in the United States; eventually, all but six states mandate immunization for all children entering kindergarten.

1995
Competing teams at two U.S. pharmaceutical companies develop vaccines for the hepatitis A virus.

1975   1985   1995   2005

1985
Reacting to the AIDS epidemic, the U.S. Food and Drug Administration places a ban on blood donations by gay men. The FDA's ban is intended to keep AIDS as well as other diseases, including hepatitis, out of the American blood supply.

1988
Michael Houghton, Qui-Lim Choo, and George Kuo, biochemists for Chrion Corporation, identify the hepatitis C virus by studying its genetic composition.

2004
Civil war in Sudan forces some 2 million residents of the Darfur region to flee to refugee camps, where an epidemic of hepatitis E afflicts some 1,700 people a month.

2006
American Red Cross calls on the FDA to rescind its policy banning blood donations by gay men.

2007
CDC reports that the infection rate for hepatitis A has fallen to its lowest level in 40 years.

Related Organizations

AABB

8101 Glenbrook Rd.

Bethesda, MD 20814-2749

phone: (301) 907-6977 • fax: (301) 907-6895

e-mail: aabb@aabb.org • Web site: www.aabb.org

Formerly known as the American Association of Blood Banks, the organization represents some 2,000 hospitals, blood donation agencies, laboratories, and other groups involved in acquiring and dispensing blood for transfusions during surgeries and other medical procedures. AABB also tracks the availability of blood in the United States and takes positions on a number of issues related to the blood supply. AABB opposes the FDA ban on blood donated by gay men.

American Liver Foundation

75 Maiden Ln., Suite 603

New York, NY 10038

phone: (212) 668-1000 • fax: (212) 483-8179

Web site: www.liverfoundation.org

Established in 1976, the American Liver Foundation promotes liver health in the United States and funds research into liver disease. Visitors to the organization's Web site can find many resources about hepatitis as well as liver transplants and view an online video of singer Naomi Judd discussing how hepatitis C affected her life.

American Medical Association (AMA)

515 N. State St.

Chicago, IL 60610

phone: (800) 621-8335

Web site: www.ama-assn.org

The national organization representing American physicians takes positions on a number of public health issues, including immunizations. In 2007 the AMA recommended broadening immunizations for hepatitis B to include not only children entering kindergarten, but also all infants, teens, military recruits, college and technical school students, and students entering medical schools. Visitors to the organization's Web site can find many articles, essays, and reports on hepatitis.

GAVI Alliance

1776 I St. NW, Suite 600

Washington, DC 20006

phone: (202) 478-1050 • fax: (202) 478-1060

Web site: www.gavialliance.org

Formerly known as the Global Alliance for Vaccines and Immunization, GAVI Alliance is a consortium of international governments and private foundations that provide immunizations to people in developing nations. A major donor to the alliance is the Bill & Melinda Gates Foundation, the philanthropic organization established by the founder of Microsoft and his wife. Since 2000, GAVI Alliance has provided hepatitis B vaccines to some 126 million children. Visitors to the organization's Web site can find reports on each country served by GAVI and learn how effective the group's work has been.

Hepatitis B Foundation

3805 Old Easton Rd.

Doylestown, PA 18902

phone: (215) 489-4900 • fax: (215) 489-4313

e-mail: info@hepb.org • Web site: www.hepb.org

The Hepatitis B Foundation helps raise money for hepatitis B research and provides support for sufferers of the disease. Established in 1991, a founding member of the organization's medical and advisory board was biochemist Baruch S. Blumberg, who won the Nobel Prize for his research that led to development of the hepatitis B vaccine. Visitors to the site can find a brief biography of Blumberg as well as the story of how he discovered the Australia antigen.

Hepatitis Foundation International

504 Blick Dr.

Silver Spring, MD 20904

phone: (800) 891-0707 • fax: (301) 622-4702

e-mail: HFI@comcast.net • Web site: www.hepfi.org

The foundation provides a number of services to hepatitis victims, including a directory of support groups, telephone hotline, public education programs, and support for hepatitis research. Visitors to the organization's Web site can find information on current research, including new antiviral drugs that are being tested in clinical trials as well as other developments in hepatitis research.

National Institutes of Health (NIH)

9000 Rockville Pike

Bethesda, MD 20892

phone: (301) 496-4000

e-mail: nihinfo@od.nih.gov • Web site: www.nih.gov

The National Institutes of Health is the chief funding arm of the federal government for medical research. Many resources about all forms of hepatitis are available on the agency's Web site, including downloadable versions of the publications *Viral Hepatitis A to E and Beyond*, *Autoimmune Hepatitis*, and *What I Need to Know About Hepatitis A*, *What I Need to Know About Hepatitis B*, and *What I Need to Know About Hepatitis C.*

U.S. Centers for Disease Control and Prevention (CDC)

Office of Communication

Building 16, D-42

1600 Clifton Rd. NE

Atlanta, GA 30333

phone: (800) 311-3435

e-mail: cdcinfo@cdc.gov • Web site: www.cdc.gov

The federal government's chief public health agency tracks infectious diseases in America. Numerous reports and studies on all forms of hepatitis and related issues are available on the CDC's Web site.

U.S. Food and Drug Administration (FDA)

5600 Fishers Ln.

Rockville, MD 20857-0001

phone: (888) 463-6332

Web site: www.fda.gov

The federal agency is charged with ensuring that the nation's food supply is produced, transported, stored, and sold in sanitary conditions to prevent the spread of food-borne diseases such as hepatitis A. Visitors to the agency's Web site can learn about hepatitis A by accessing the FDA's "Bad Bug Book." The FDA's position opposing blood donations by gay men can also be read on the Web site.

U.S. National Center for Health Statistics

3311 Toledo Rd.

Hyattsville, MD 20782

phone: (800) 232-4636

e-mail: nchsquery@cdc.gov • Web site: www.cdc.gov

Part of the CDC, the center compiles statistics and reports on hepatitis and many other diseases and health-related topics. The report *Health,*

United States 2007, which includes statistics on diseases common in the United States, can be downloaded from the center's Web site.

World Health Organization (WHO)

Ave. Appia 20, CH-1211

Geneva 27, Switzerland

phone: +41 22 791 2111 • fax: +41 22 791 3111

e-mail: info@who.int • Web site: www.who.int

WHO is the public health arm of the United Nations. The agency tracks the spread of diseases across the globe and responds to many public health crises, such as rushing vaccines to impoverished or war-torn nations during epidemics. Visitors to the organization's Web site can download many reports about the worldwide hepatitis situation.

For Further Research

Books

James L. Achord, *Understanding Hepatitis*. Jackson: University Press of Mississippi, 2002.

Baruch S. Blumberg, *Hepatitis B: The Hunt for a Killer Virus*. Princeton, NJ: Princeton University Press, 2002.

Sanjiv Chopra, *Dr. Sanjiv Chopra's Liver Book*. New York: Pocket Books, 2001.

Sabrina D. Craigo and Emily R. Baker, *Medical Complications in Pregnancy*. New York: McGraw-Hill, 2005.

Margaret C. Fisher, ed., *Immunizations & Infectious Diseases*. Elk Grove Village, IL: American Academy of Pediatrics, 2006.

Laurie Garrett, *The Coming Plague: Newly Emerging Diseases in a World Out of Balance*. New York: Farrar, Straus & Giroux, 1994.

John King, ed., *Mayo Clinic on Digestive Health*. Rochester, MN: Mayo Clinic Health Information, 2004.

Arien Mack, ed., *In Time of Plague: The History and Social Consequences of Lethal Epidemic Disease*. New York: New York University Press, 1991.

Melissa Palmer, *Melissa Palmer's Guide to Hepatitis Liver Disease*. Garden City Park, NY: Avery, 2000.

David Rifkin and Geraldine L. Freeman, *The Nobel Prize Winning Discoveries in Infectious Diseases*. London: Elsevier, 2005.

Periodicals

Ginny Clark, "Beating a Stigma and Staying Alive," *Glasgow Herald*, August 29, 2007.

Geoffrey Cowley, Karen Springen, Anne Underwood, Nadine Joseph, Joan Raymond, and John Horn, "Hepatitis C: The Insidious Spread of a Killer Virus," *Newsweek*, April 22, 2002.

Paul Davies, "Long-Dormant Threat Surfaces: Deaths from Hepatitis C Are Expected to Jump," *Wall Street Journal*, May 31, 2005.

Economist, "Needles and Haystacks," November 1, 2003.

Anita Elash, "Hepatitis: Silent Predator," *Maclean's*, July 1, 1997.

Stanley M. Finger, "Families in Crisis," *Scientist*, May 2007.

Olivia Holcombe, "The Secret Assassin," *Daily Mail* (London), February 20, 2007.

Carolyn Hughes, "Living with Hepatitis C," *Saturday Evening Post*, September/October 1999.

Corey Kilgannon, "So Many Hepatitis Cases, So Many Cures," *New York Times*, May 13, 2006.

Janet Kinosian, "Naomi Judd: Brave Battle Against Hepatitis C," *Saturday Evening Post*, January/February 1996.

Lorraine Kreahling, "The Peril of Needles to the Body," *New York Times*, February 1, 2005.

William Little, "The Day the Music Stopped," *Times* (London), March 16, 2005.

Anita Manning, "Hepatitis, 'the Silent Killer,' Driven Out of the Shadows; New Medications, Research Bring Hope, Treatment, Even Cures," *USA Today*, January 23, 2006.

Justin Martin, "Hepatitis C, the Quiet Epidemic," *Fortune*, August 7, 1995.

Martha Mendoza, "Prisons Breed Hepatitis C Victims, Nobody Knows How Many Inmates Have the Disease, Which Can Be Treated," *Pittsburgh Post-Gazette*, Associated Press, March 18, 2007.

Mitzi Miller, "A Lesson Before Dying," *Essence*, August 2007.

Michelle Mueller, "Hepatitis C: The Silent Epidemic," *Current Health 2*, January 2004.

Joyce Howard Price, "Disease, Unwanted Import," *Washington Times*, February 13, 2005.

Betsy Querna, "Emerging Epidemic," *U.S. News & World Report*, March 13, 2006.

Nancy Shute, E.F. Licking, and Stacey Schultz, "Hepatitis C: A Silent Killer," *U.S. News & World Report*, June 22, 1998.

Edna Strauss and Maria Christina Dias Teixeira, "Quality of Life in Hepatitis C," *Liver International*, 2006.

Anaya Toney and Richard Raymond, "Hepatitis A: A Preventable Threat to Hispanics," *Hispanic*, November 1998.

Kai Wright, "Prison Outbreak: An Epidemic of Hepatitis C," *Progressive*, March 2006.

Internet Sources

CNN.com/health, "Researchers Clone Pigs," August 16, 2000. http://archives/cnn.com/2000/HEALTH/08/16/pig.clones.

CNN.com, "Terror Bust; Border Insecurity; Political Climate; Ocean Pollution; Illegal Immigrants and Disease; Outsourcing Not Worth It?" *Lou Dobbs Tonight*, June 8, 2005. http://transcripts.cnn.com/TRANSCRIPTS/0506/08/ldt.01.html.

National Academy of Sciences, "The Hepatitis B Story," *Beyond Discovery*, February 2000. www.beyonddiscovery.org/content/view.article.asp?a=265.

Science Daily, "Science Turns Mouse into Factory for Human Liver Cells," August 10, 2007. www.sciencedaily.com/releases/2007/08/070809172151.htm.

————, "Who Will Recover Spontaneously from Hepatitis C Virus Infection?" August 29, 2007. www.sciencedaily.com/releases/2007/08/070829102044.htm.

Stephen Steele, "In Northeastern Chad's Heat and Rain, Refugee Graves Are Added Daily," *Catholic News Service*, September 2, 2004. http://catholicnews.com/data/stories/cns/0404837.htm.

Sudan Tribune, "Sharp Jump in Hepatitis E Cases in Darfur: WHO," August 28, 2004. www.sudantribune.com/spip.php?article5042.

Source Notes

Overview

1. Quoted in Nancy Shute, E.F. Licking, and Stacey Schultz, "Hepatitis C: A Silent Killer," *U.S. News & World Report*, June 22, 1998, p. 60.
2. James L. Achord, *Understanding Hepatitis.* Jackson: University Press of Mississippi, 2002, p 38.
3. Quoted in *Daily Times* (Lahore, Pakistan), "Our 10 Million Hepatitis Patients Could Create an Epidemic: Experts," July 22, 2007. www.daily times.com.
4. Quoted in Geoffrey Cowley et al., "Hepatiris C: The Insidious Spread of a Killer Virus," *Newsweek*, April 22, 2002, p. 46.
5. Quoted in Janet Kinosian, "Naomi Judd: Brave Battle Against Hepatitis C," *Saturday Evening Post*, January/February 1996, p. 36.
6. Edna Strauss and Maria Christina Dias Teixeira, "Quality of Life in Hepatitis C," *Liver International*, 2006, p. 757.
7. Quoted in Lorraine Kreahling, "The Perils of Needles to the Body," *New York Times*, February 1, 2005, p. F-5.

How Does Hepatitis Affect People?

8. Quoted in William Little, "The Day the Music Stopped," *Times* (London), March 16, 2005. www.timesonline.co.uk.
9. Quoted in Cowley et al., "Hepatitis C: The Insidious Spread of a Killer Virus," p. 46.
10. Achord, *Understanding Hepatitis*, p. 30.
11. Quoted in Olivia Holcombe, "The Secret Assassin," *Daily Mail* (London), February 20, 2007, p. 51.
12. Quoted in Betsy Querna, "Emerging Epidemic," *U.S. News & World Report*, March 13, 2006, p. 60.
13. Quoted in Anita Elash, "Hepatitis: Silent Predator," *Maclean's*, July 1, 1997, p. 98.

How Prevalent Is Hepatitis?

14. Quoted in John Gallagher, "The Next Epidemic? Gays and Hepatitis," *Advocate*, April 28, 1998.
15. Quoted in Carla K. Johnson, "Many States Don't Vaccinate Underinsured Children," *Columbus (OH) Dispatch*, Associated Press, August 8, 2007. www.columbusdispatch.com.
16. World Health Organization, Department of Communicable Disease Surveillance and Response, *Hepatitis A*, July 2000, p. 5.
17. World Health Organization, Department of Communicable Disease Surveillance and Response, *Hepatitis B*, February 2002, p. 8.
18. World Health Organization, Department of Communicable Disease Surveillance and Response, *Hepatitis E*, December 2001, p. 4.
19. Quoted in Shute, Licking, and Schultz, "Hepatitis C: A Silent Killer," p. 60.
20. Quoted in Stephen Smith, "Hepatitis C Rises Among Young People, Massachusetts Officials Suspect Jump Tied to Drug Use," *Boston Globe*, May 8, 2007. www.boston.com.

What Are the Social Impacts of Hepatitis?

21. Quoted in Ginny Clark, "Beating a Stigma and Staying Alive," *Glasgow Herald*, August 29, 2007.
22. Strauss and Teixeira, "Quality of Life in Hepatitis C." www.theherald.co.uk.

23. Quoted in Patricia Anstett, "Naomi Judd Offers Hope to Those with Disease," *Detroit Free Press*, June 19, 1998.

24. Quoted in Adam Cresswell, "The Hidden Epidemic," *Australian* (Sydney), September 30, 2006.

25. Stanley M. Finger, "Families in Crisis," *Scientist*, May 2007. www.thescientist.com.

26. Quoted in David Bruce, "Parlor Protection," *Portland Oregonian*, August 30, 2006.

27. Quoted in Spike Gillespie, "Needlemania," *Texas Monthly*, September 1996, p. 78.

28. Quoted in Kai Wright, "Prison Outbreak: An Epidemic of Hepatitis C," *Progressive*, March 2006, p. 33.

29. Quoted in Martha Mendoza, "Prisons Breed Hepatitis C Victims; Nobody Knows How Many Inmates Have the Disease, Which Can Be Treated," *Pittsburgh Post-Gazette*, Associated Press, March 18, 2007, p. A-6.

30. Quoted in Joyce Howard Price, "Disease, Unwanted Import," *Washington Times*, February 13, 2005.

31. Quoted in Anaya Toney and Richard Raymond, "Hepatitis A: A Preventable Threat to Hispanics," *Hispanic*, November 1998, p. 64.

32. Quoted in *Lou Dobbs Tonight*, CNN, June 8, 2005. http://transcripts.cnn.com.

Can Hepatitis Be Prevented?

33. Quoted in Nicholas Bakalar, "Progress Is Seen Against Hepatitis," *New York Times*, March 27, 2007, p. F-6.

34. Quoted in Toney and Raymond, "Hepatitis A: A Preventable Threat to Hispanics," p. 64.

35. Quoted in *Economist*, "Needles and Haystacks," November 1, 2003, p. 75.

36. Achord, *Understanding Hepatitis*, p. 118.

37. Achord, *Understanding Hepatitis*, p. 118.

38. Quoted in Steven Bodzin, "Red Cross Eases Ban on Gay Donors," *Boston Globe*, Bloomberg News, March 18, 2006. http://boston.com.

39. Quoted in GAVI Alliance, "China Immunizes Millions of Children Against Hepatitis B in Historic Collaboration Between Government and GAVI Alliance," news release, July 25, 2006. http://gavialliance.org.

List of Illustrations

Index

About the Author

Hal Marcovitz, a writer based in Chalfont, Pennsylvania, has written more than 100 books for young adult readers. His other titles in the Compact Research series include *Meningitis* and *Phobias*.